For Madeline and Emmett, Aria and Diana

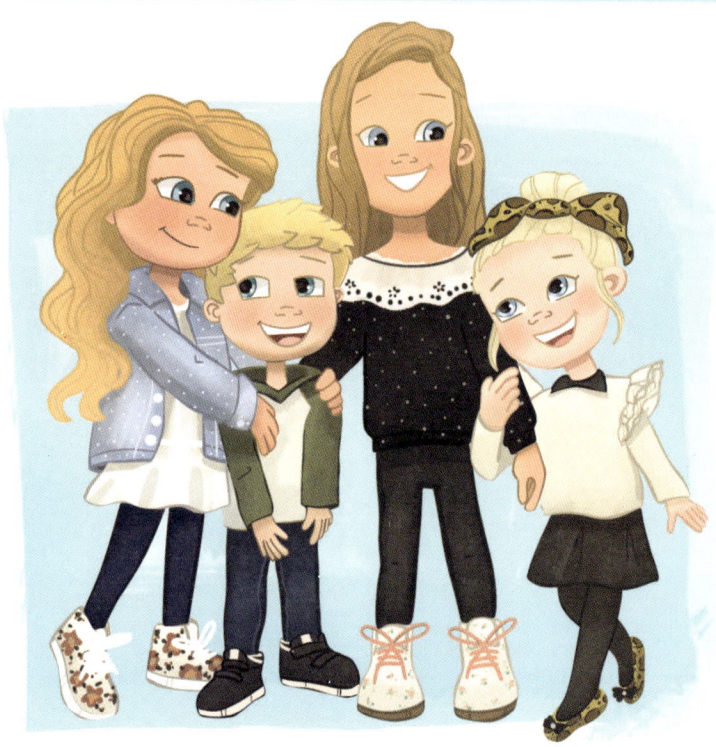

Copyright © Safely Anchored LLC
All rights reserved.
Text by Jennifer Jenkins and Samantha Paul
Illustrations by Sierra Ward

First Edition, 2021

ISBN 978-1-7369200-0-8
Library of Congress Control Number: 2021907029

Published By Safely Anchored LLC
Dayton, Ohio
Printed by Twain's Press
Printed in China

www.safelyanchored.com

Special Thanks To:

Susan and Troy Wotherspoon
Don and Carolyn Wotherspoon
John and Diane Bahme
Kelly McElhaney
Brittany A. Garcia
Kimberly
Kara and Dave Cervo
Tyler and Mishaela Wotherspoon
Will and Kristin Giddings
John and Terry Paul
Amanda Louder
The Whale Family
The Swanson Family
Cindy Madsen
JB & CN
Jessica Allred
Liz Knowles
Rebecca Martell
Katie Cross

I Know Myself

Understanding Body Science, Safety, and Self-Love

By Jennifer Jenkins and Samantha Paul
Illustrated by Sierra Ward

Safely Anchored LLC

What is an affirmation?

Positive affirmations are sentences we repeat to ourselves to make positive thought changes!

This book uses affirmations on every page to help us remember what we are learning, how great we are, and what we can do!

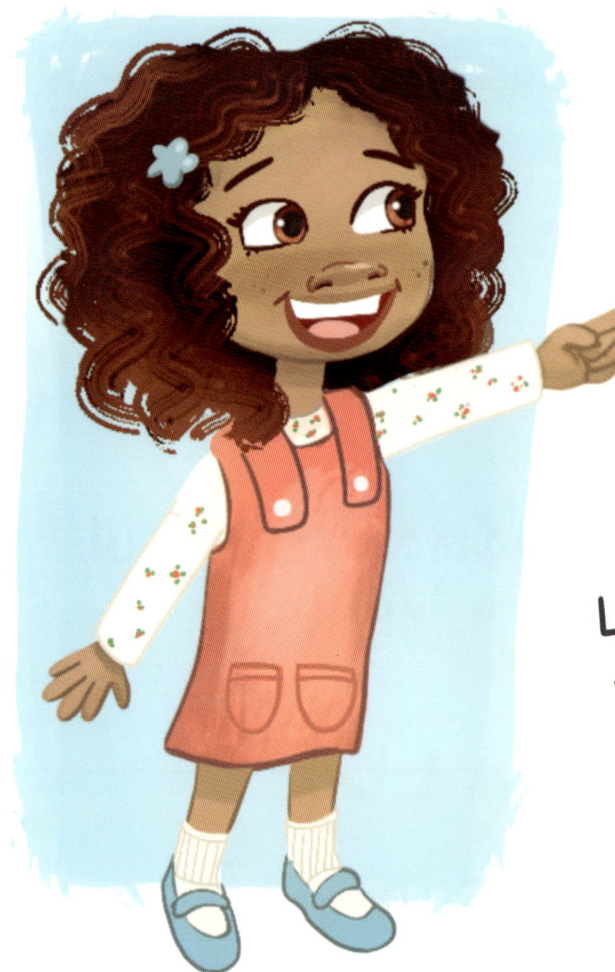

Repeat:
I know myself!

Look for the cloud on each page that gives you an affirmation to say!

Affirmations

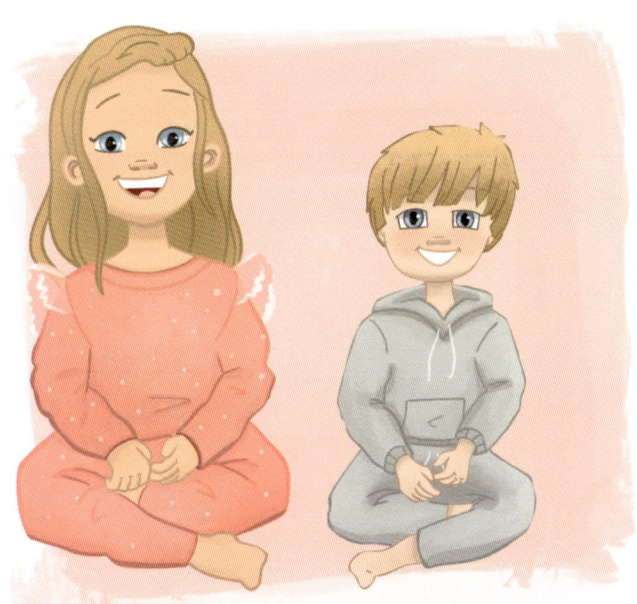

First, find any comfortable position. You can be standing, sitting, or lying down.

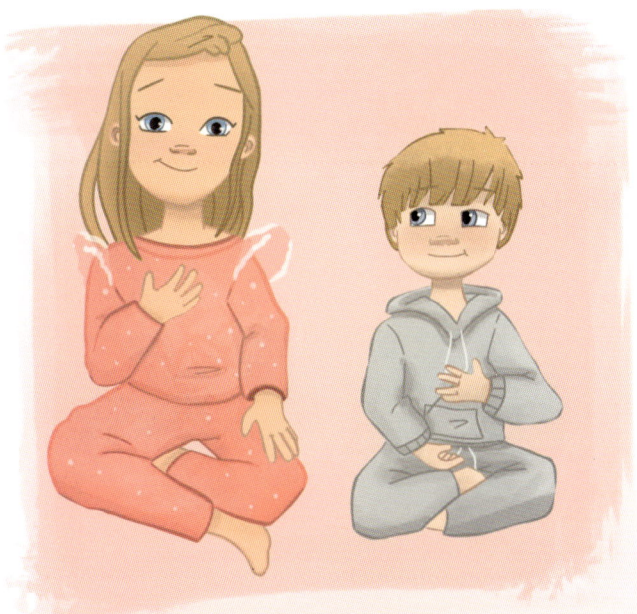

Second, place your hand on your heart.

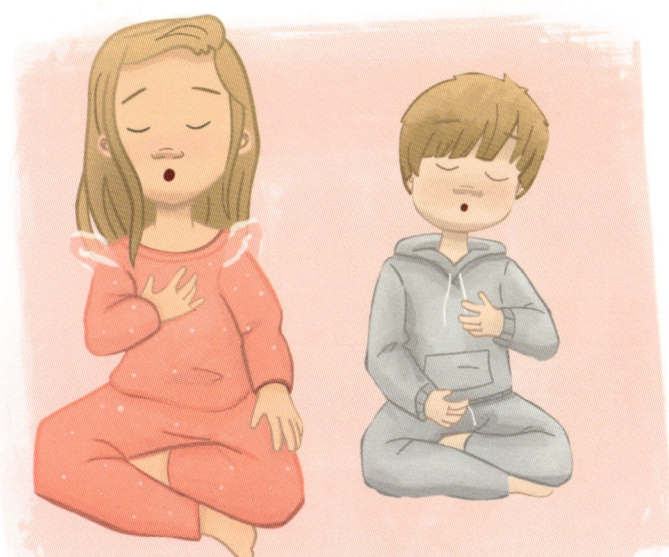

Third, take a deep breath: in through your nose and out through your mouth.

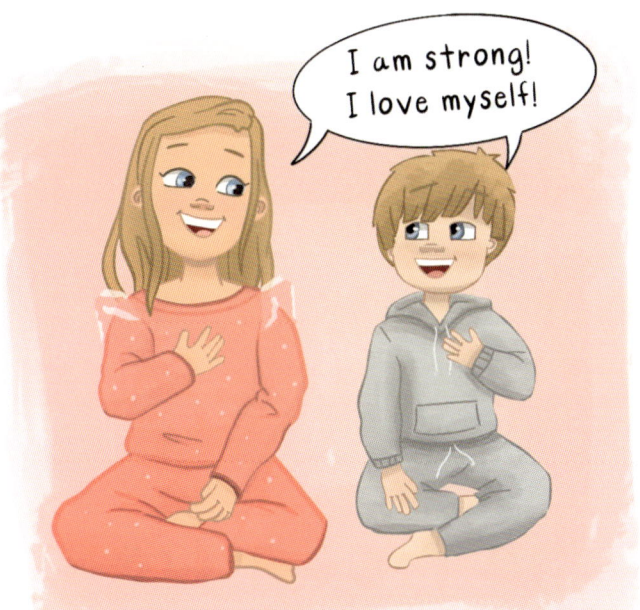

I am strong! I love myself!

Last, repeat the affirmations in the cloud on each page out loud or in your head.

We all want to be safe and feel safe.

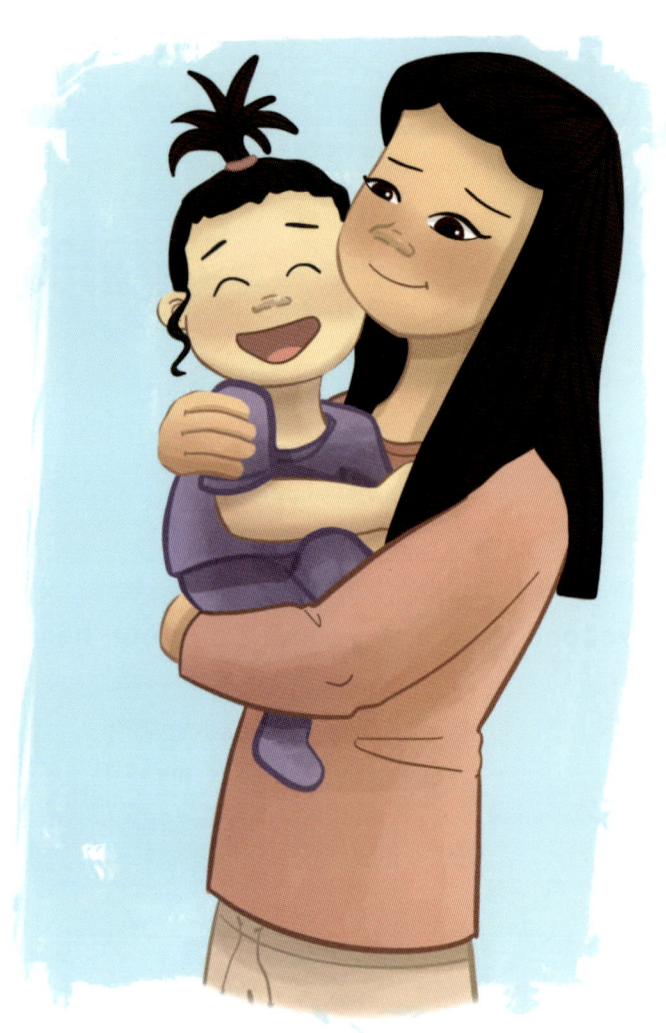

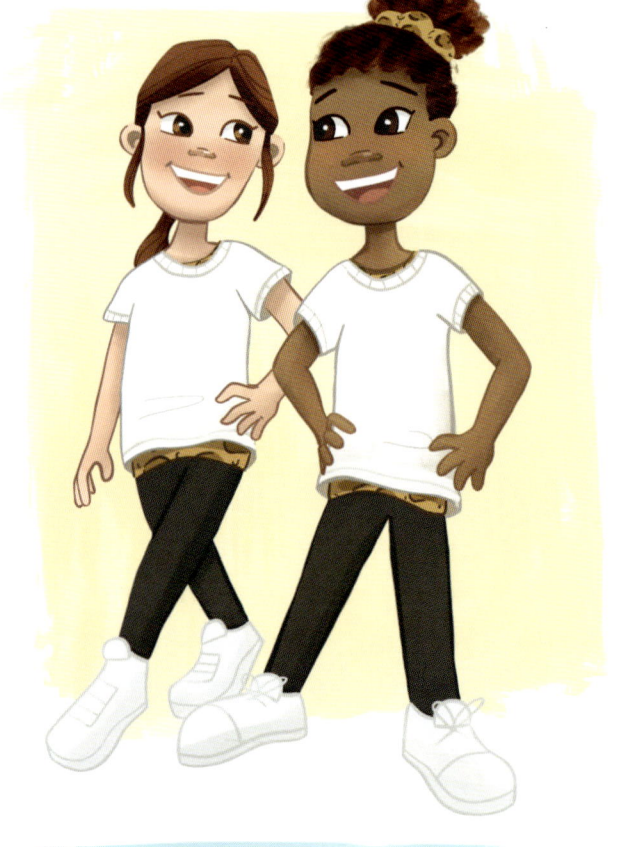

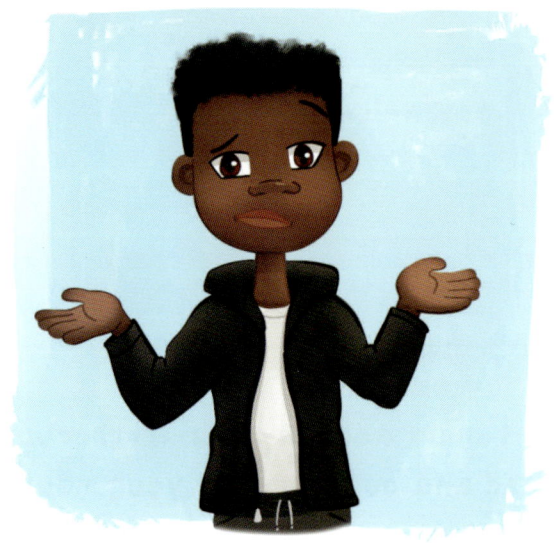

What can we do?

FIRST...

It is important to understand how your body works!

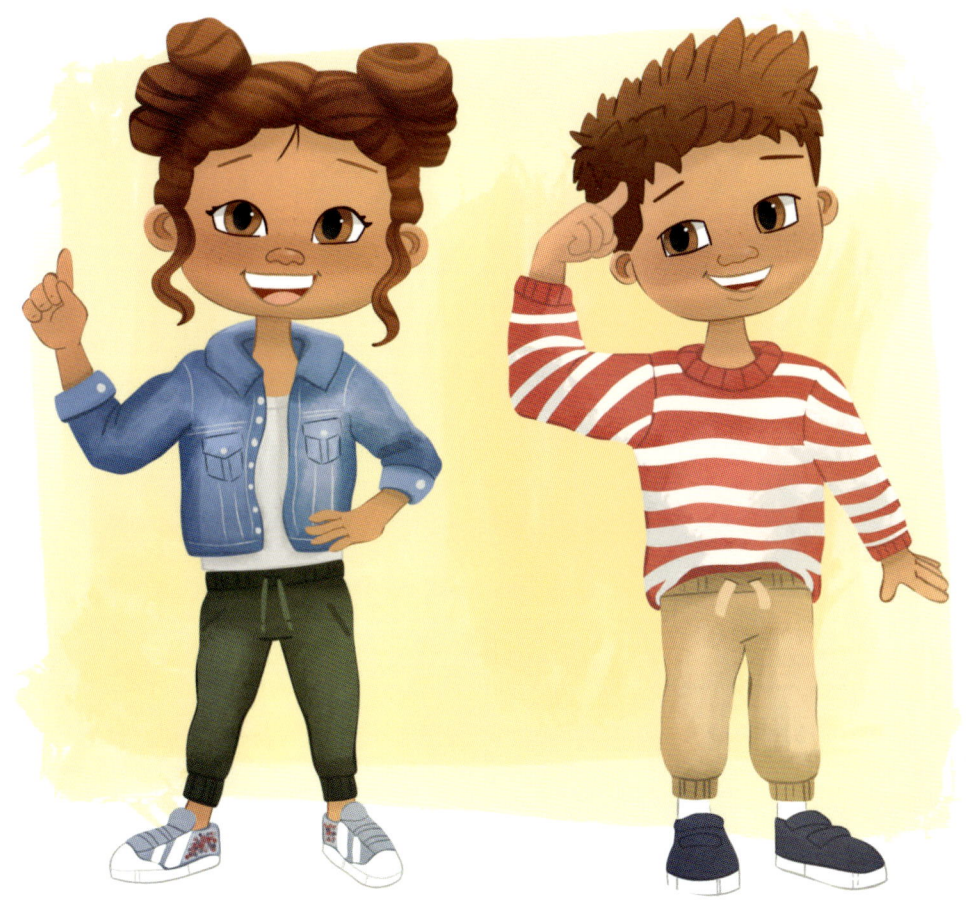

The next pages show the inside of our body and how babies grow, are born, and thrive.

Look inside your body!

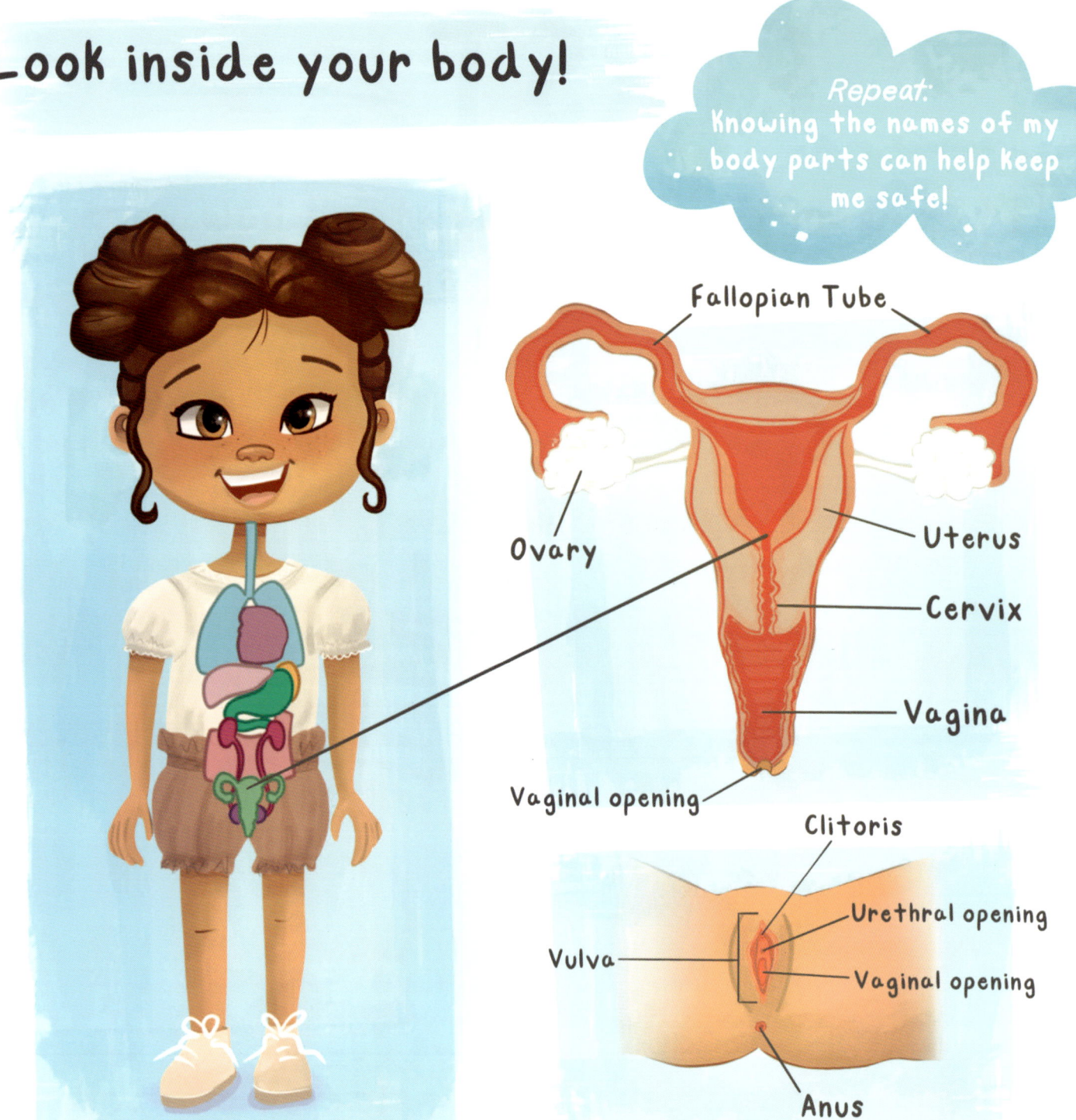

Repeat:
Knowing the names of my body parts can help keep me safe!

Fallopian Tube

Ovary

Uterus

Cervix

Vagina

Vaginal opening

Clitoris

Vulva

Urethral opening

Vaginal opening

Anus

Girls have body parts that are unique to them!

Using the correct names for your body parts helps keep you safe!

Bladder

Urethra

Penis

Testicle

Scrotum

Bladder

Testicle

Penis

Urethra

Glans

Foreskin

Circumcised

Uncircumcised

Boys have body parts that are unique to them!

We are all special and unique!
We come from something so small!

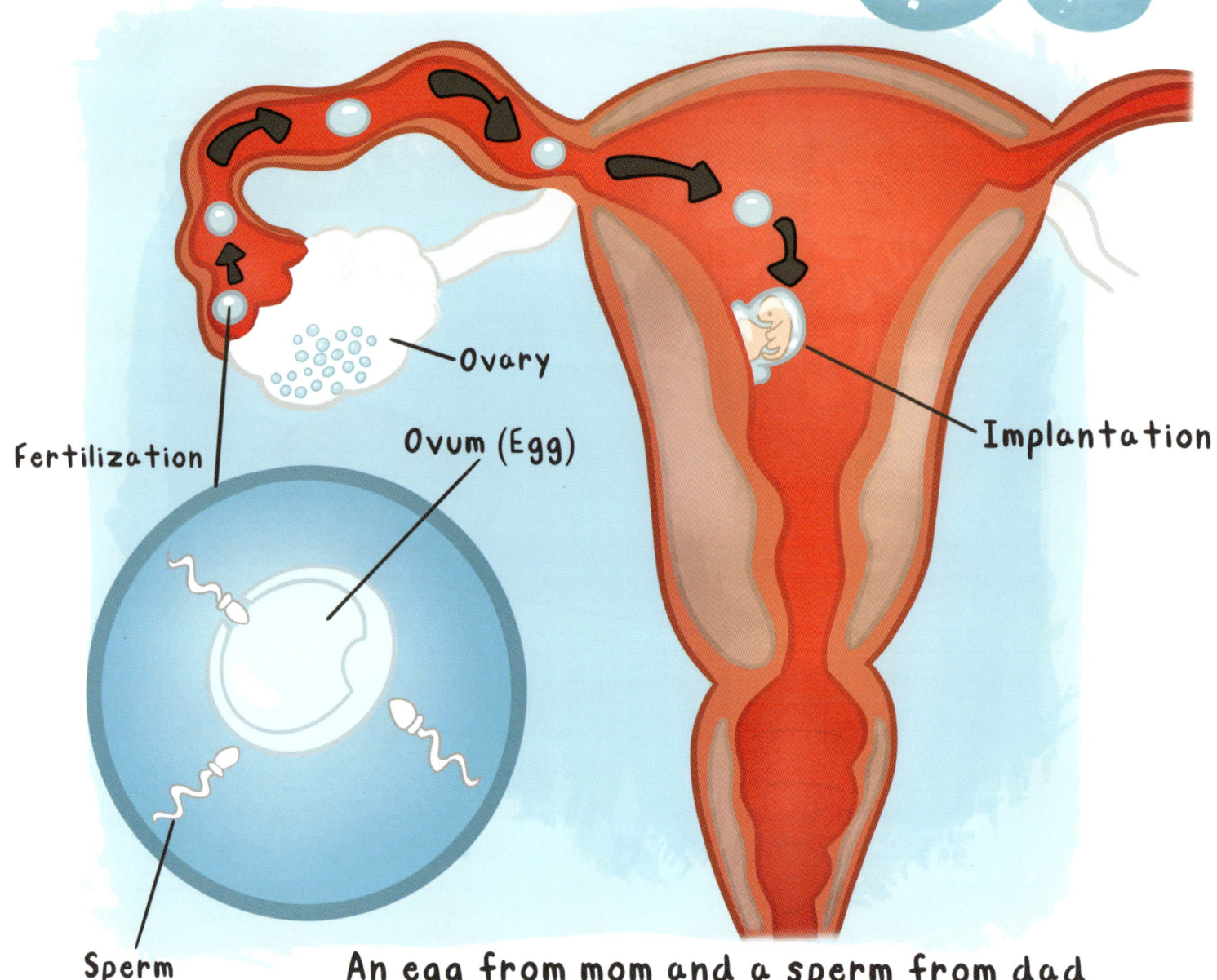

Ovary

Fertilization

Ovum (Egg)

Implantation

Sperm

An egg from mom and a sperm from dad
met and created you!

Look at how babies grow!

Repeat:
I grow everyday!

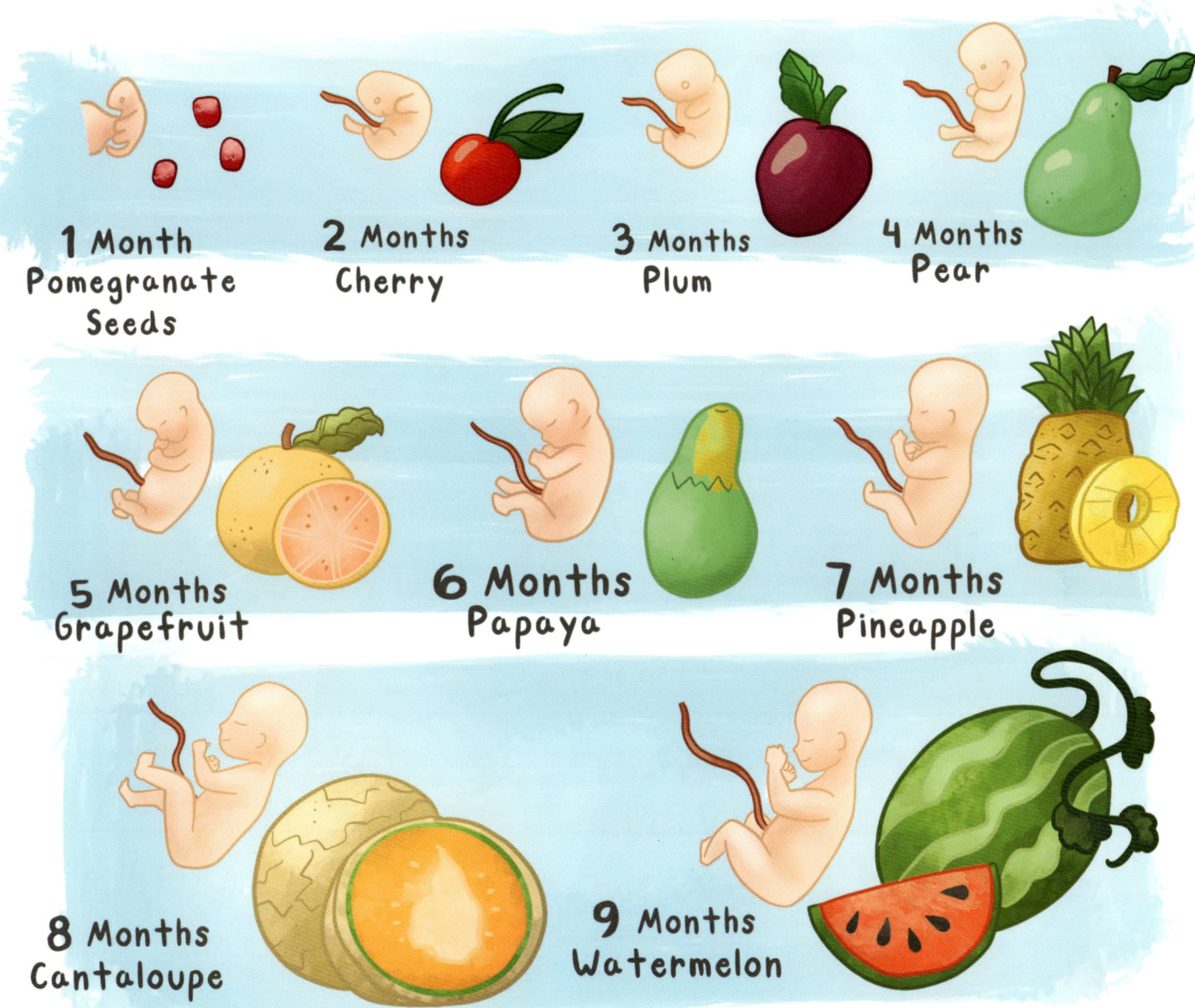

1 Month
Pomegranate
Seeds

2 Months
Cherry

3 Months
Plum

4 Months
Pear

5 Months
Grapefruit

6 Months
Papaya

7 Months
Pineapple

8 Months
Cantaloupe

9 Months
Watermelon

A woman's body makes room for a baby to grow until the baby is ready to be born and meet the world!

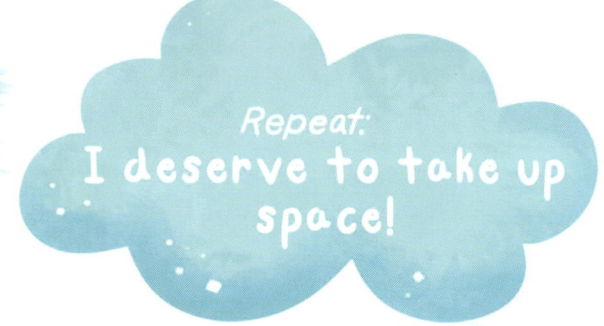
Repeat:
I deserve to take up space!

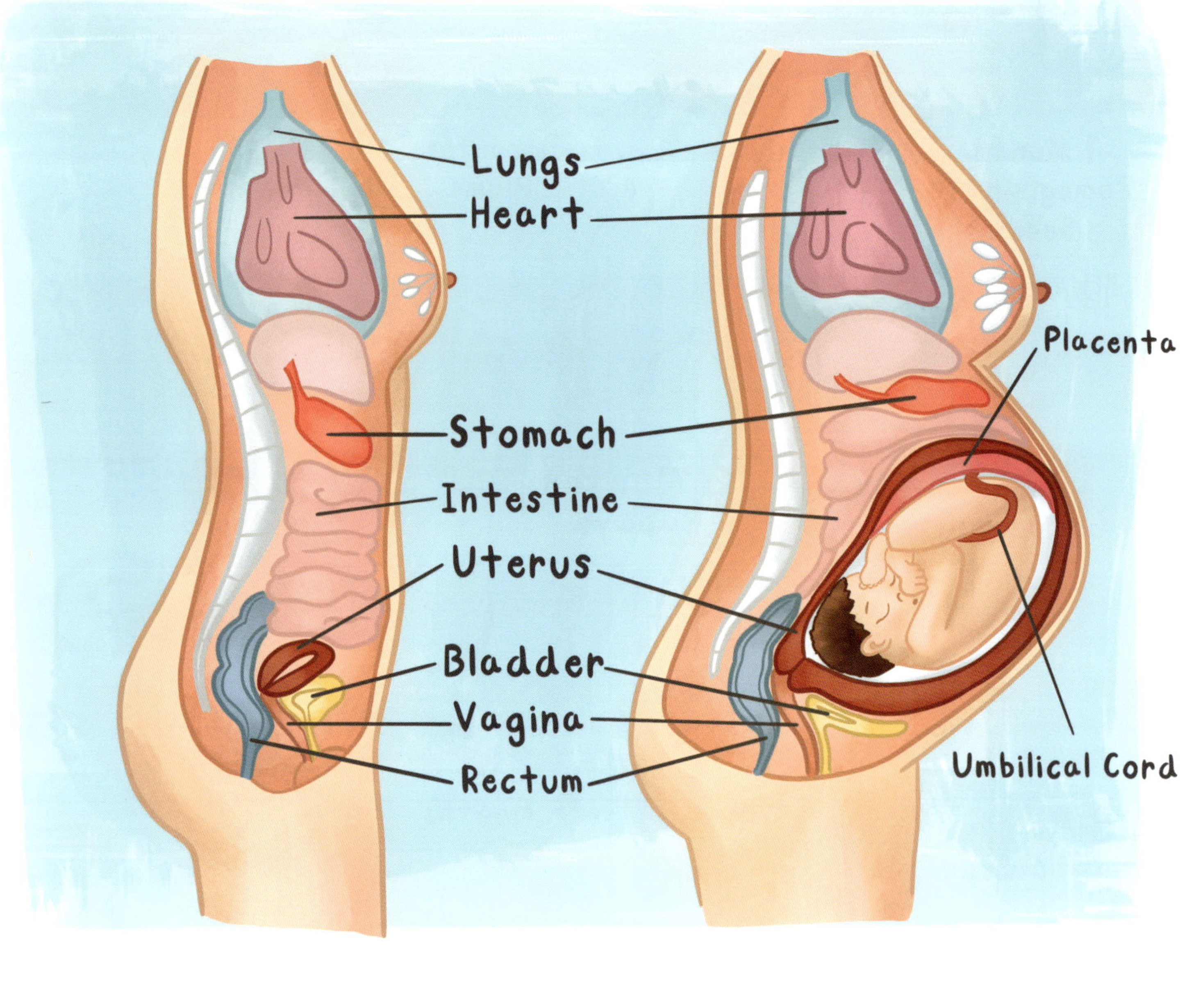

Lungs

Heart

Placenta

Stomach

Intestine

Uterus

Bladder

Vagina

Rectum

Umbilical Cord

Babies are born in different ways!

Vaginal Birth

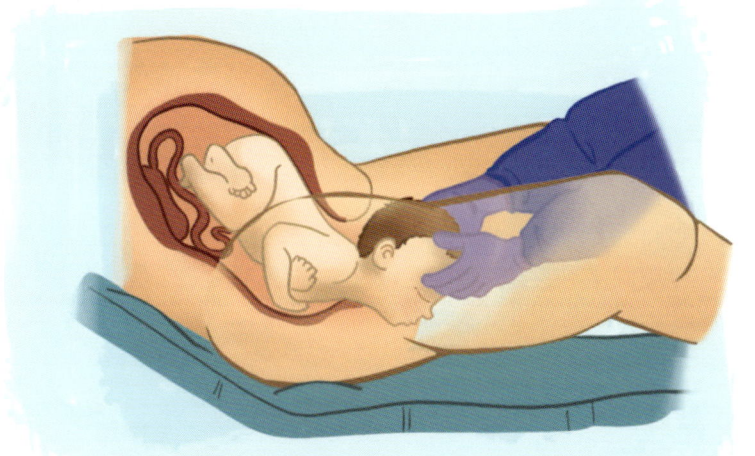
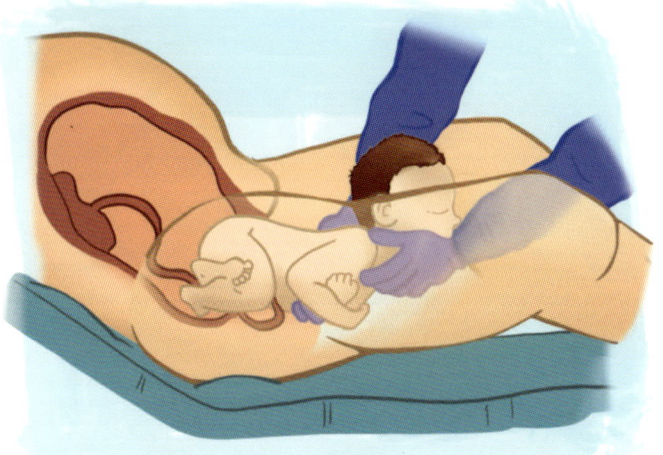

C Section

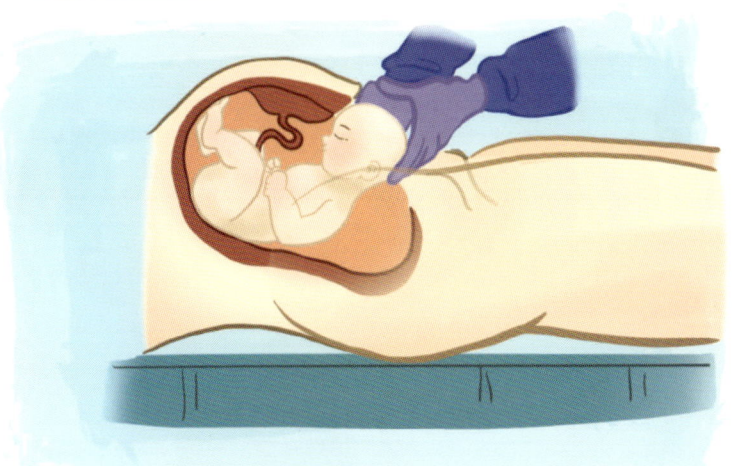
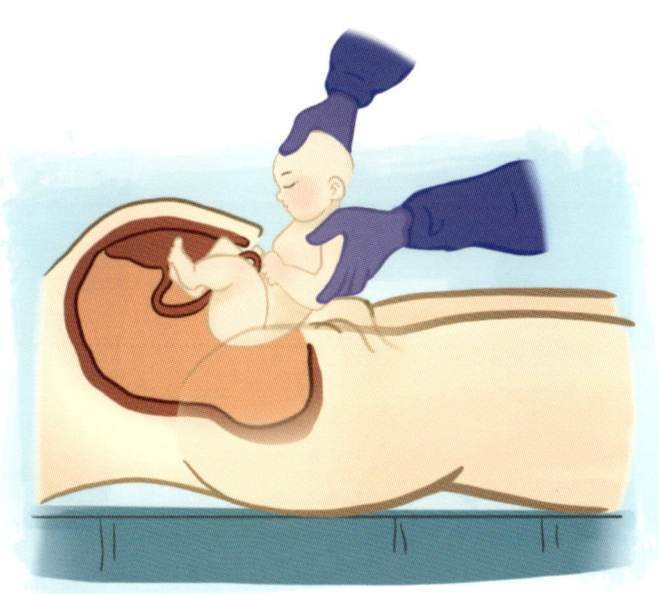

Babies need to eat so they can grow!
Look at all the ways to keep baby
fed!

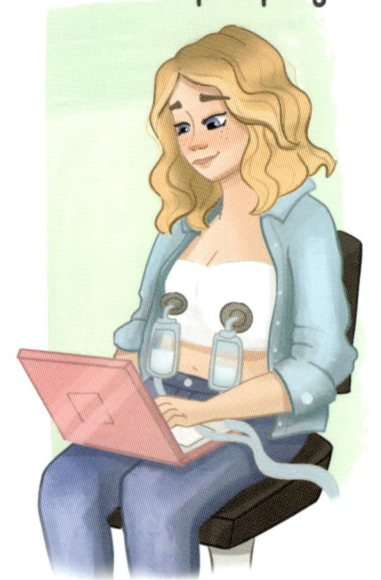

Repeat:
Nourishing my body
helps me grow!

Breast pumping

Breast Feeding

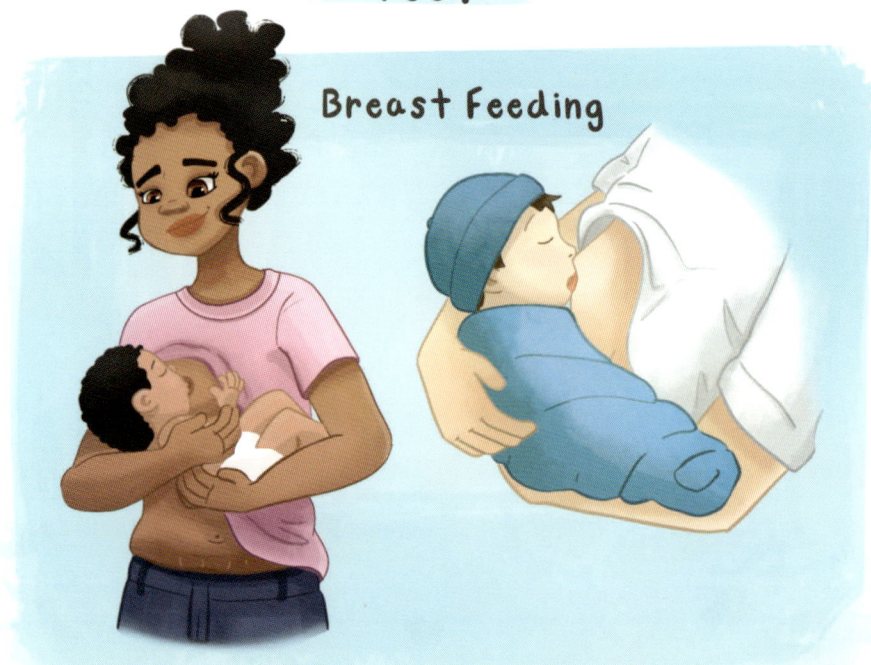

Bottle Feeding

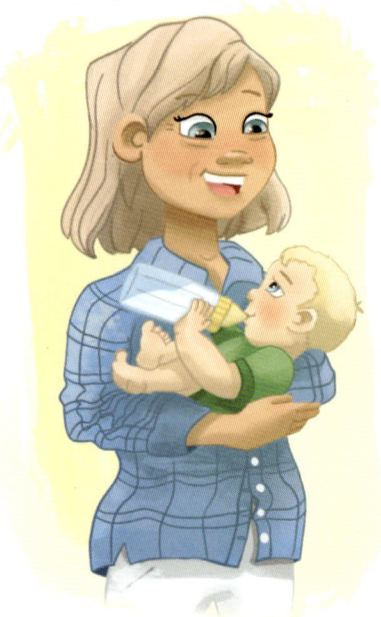

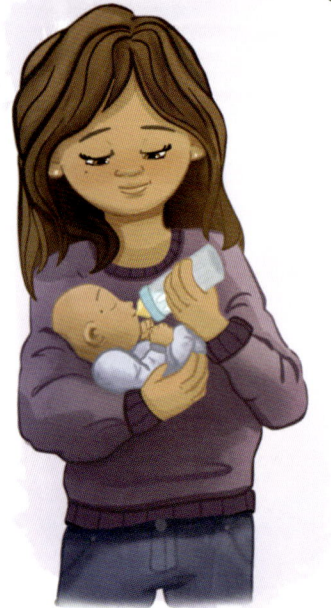

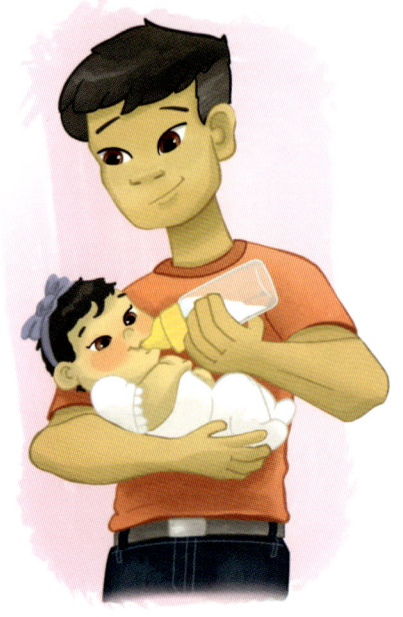

Babies have needs and need to be cared for and protected, just like us!

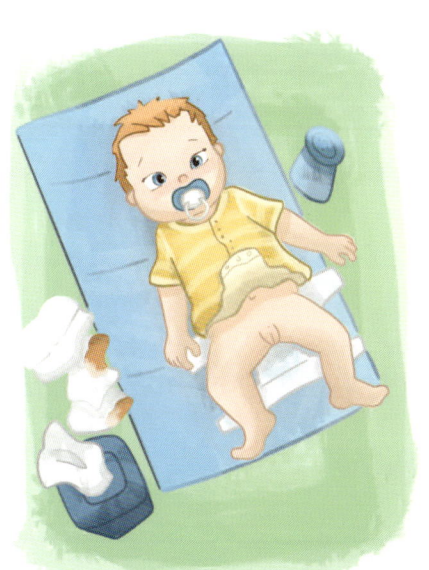
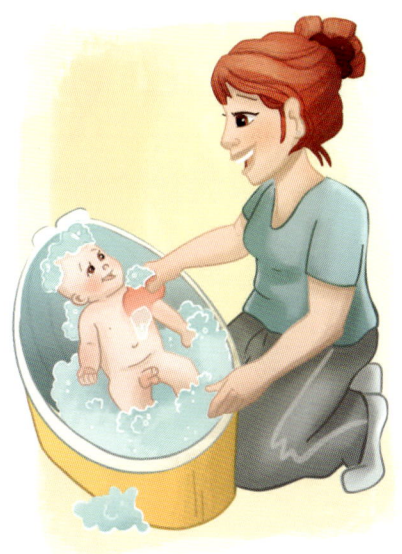
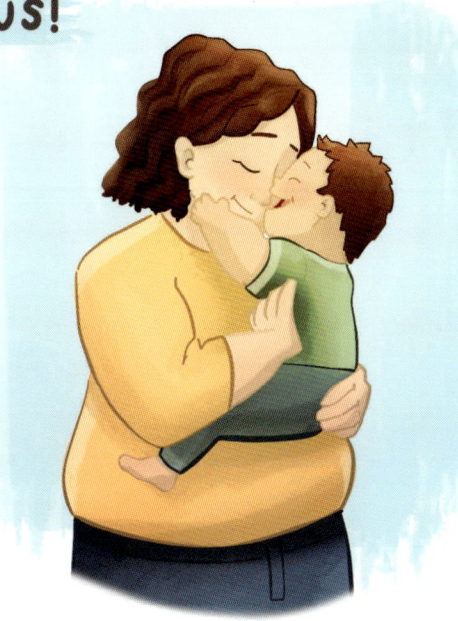

Babies also need clean diapers, baths, sleep, hugs, love, and attention!

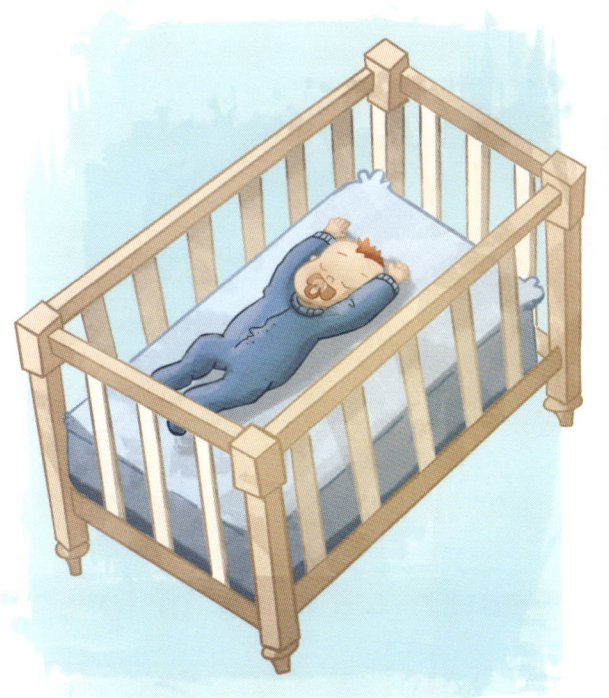
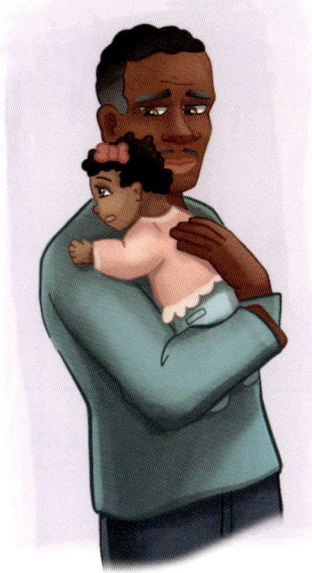
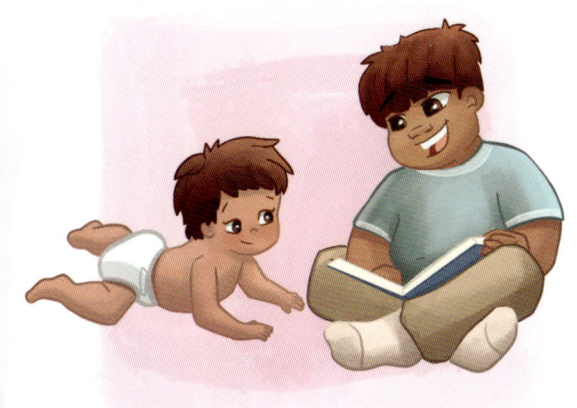

Repeat:
Paying attention to my needs is important!

SECOND...

It is important to know how to protect our bodies!

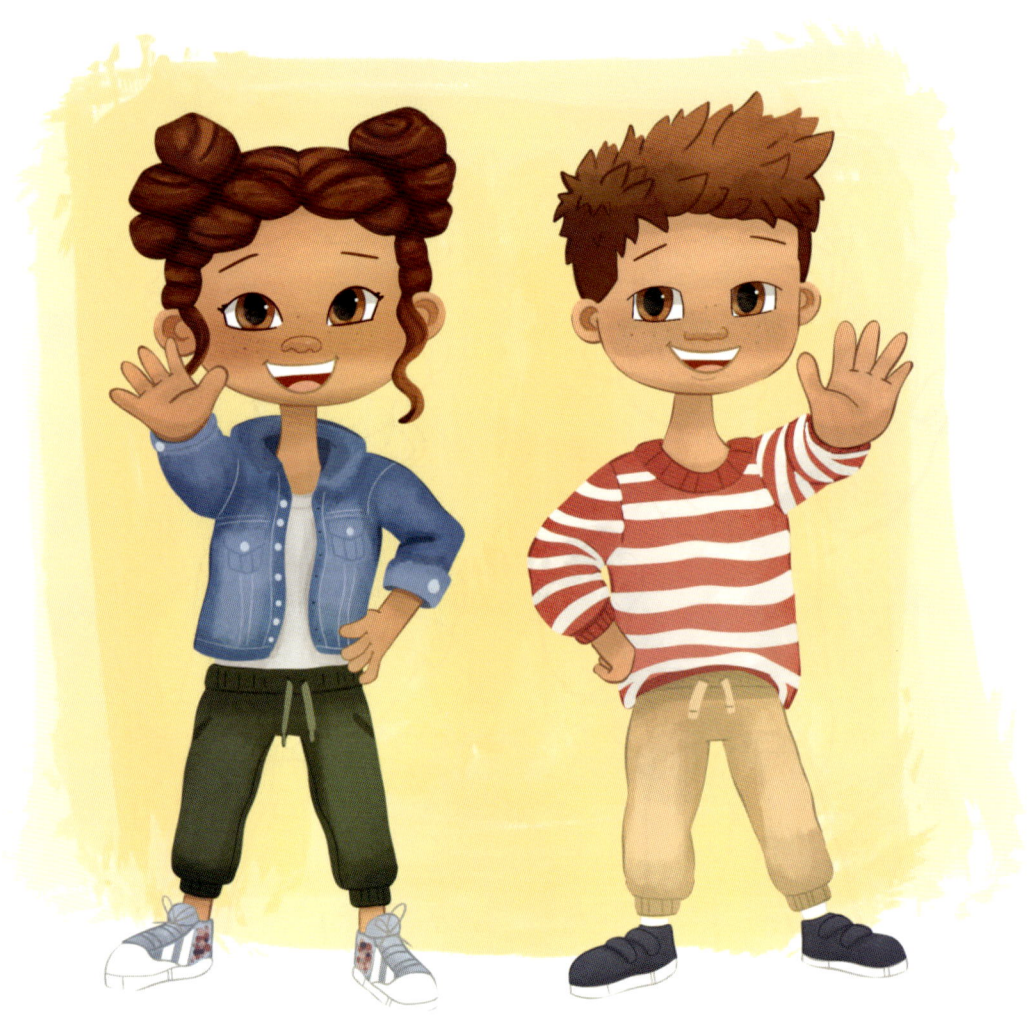

The next pages show when to let safe adults help and that our bodies and voices belong to us.

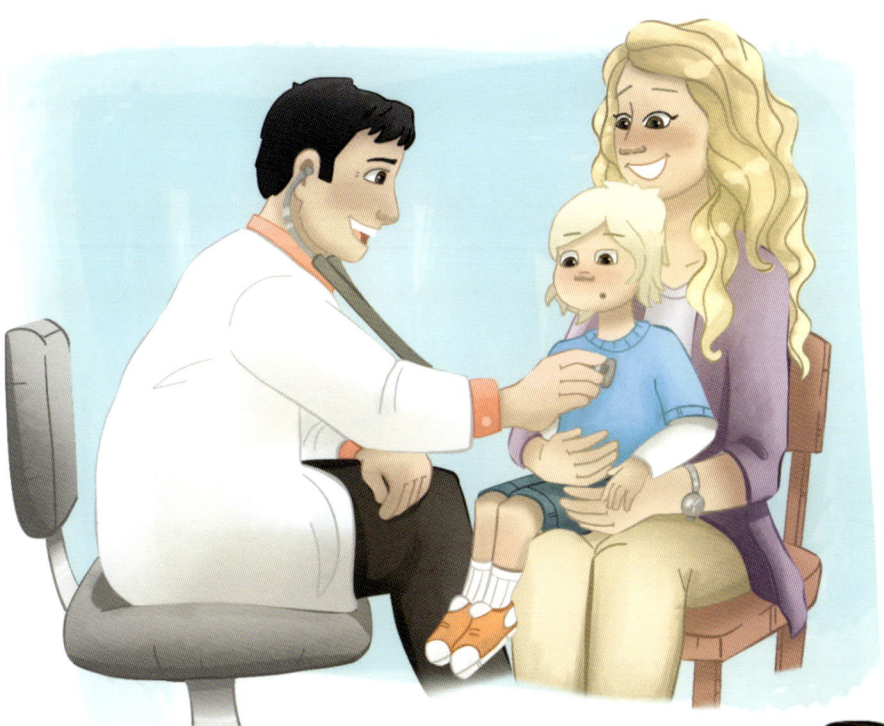

At the doctor

There are safe adults we trust that are here to help us with certain needs.

Repeat:
Adults are here to help when I need it!

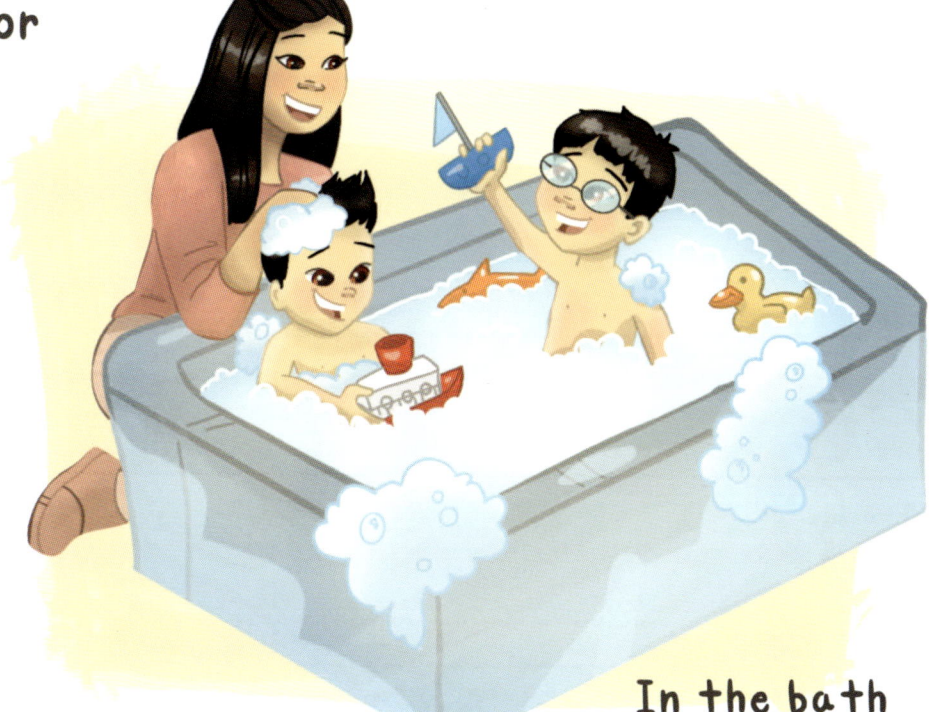

In the bath

Your body belongs to you! Everyone else's body belongs to them!

Repeat:
My body belongs to me! I respect my body!

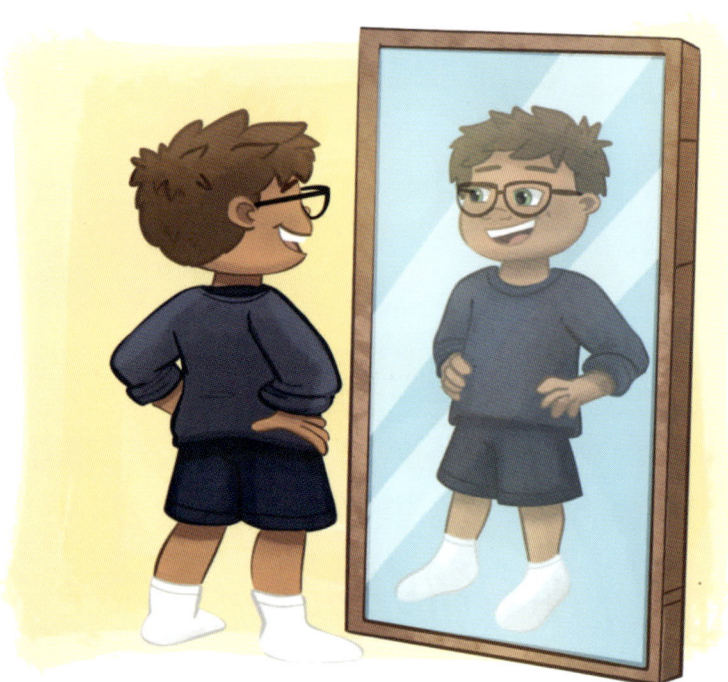

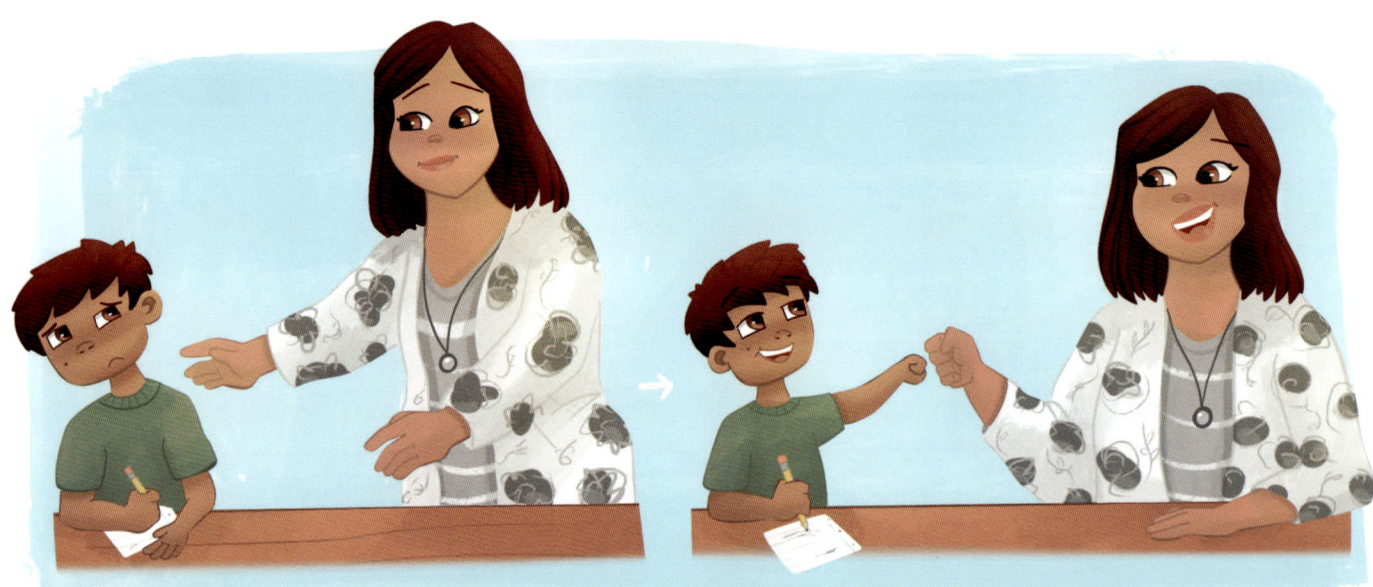

It's okay to not want to be touched or hugged, even by adults you know!

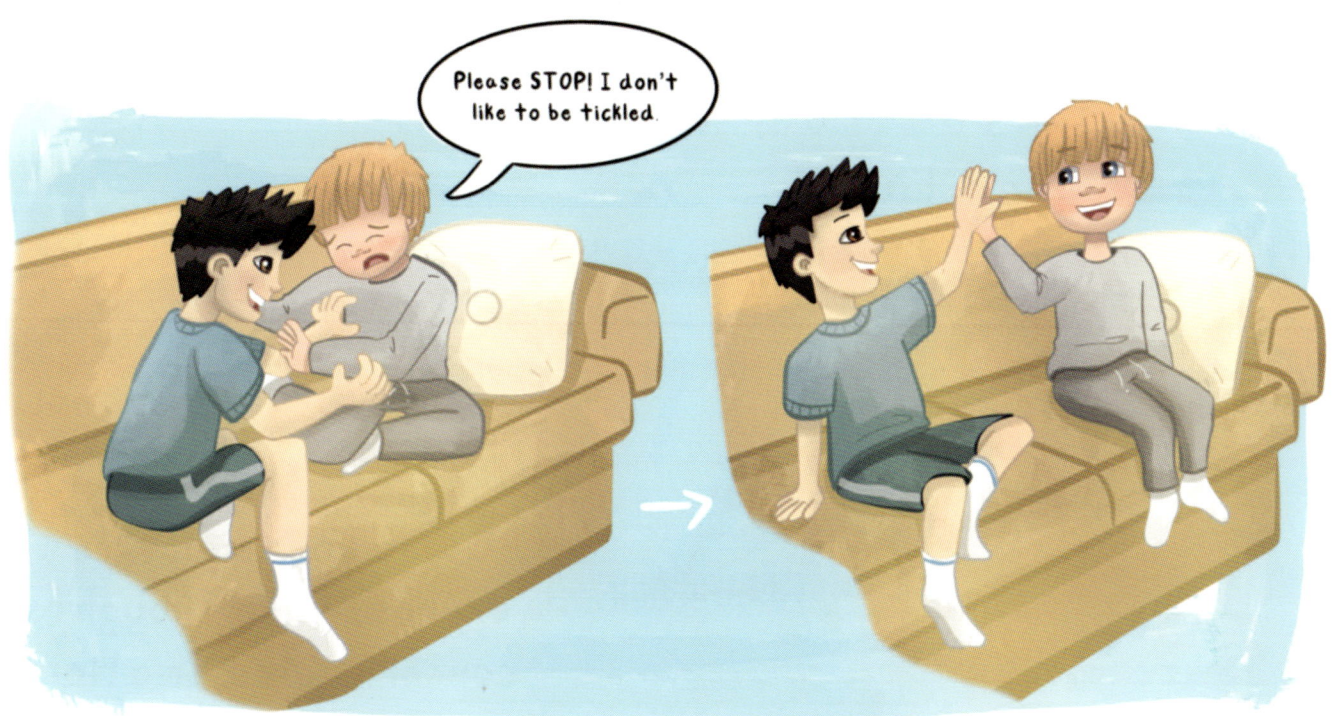

It's important to respect other people's bodies and boundaries! We all need boundaries so we can show up safely and confidently in our lives! Boundaries are like invisible lines that we don't cross or let others cross.

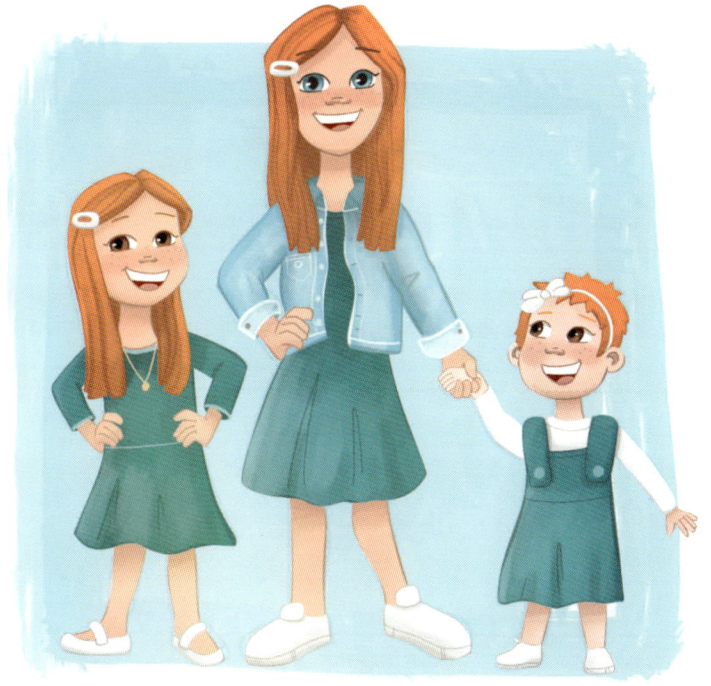

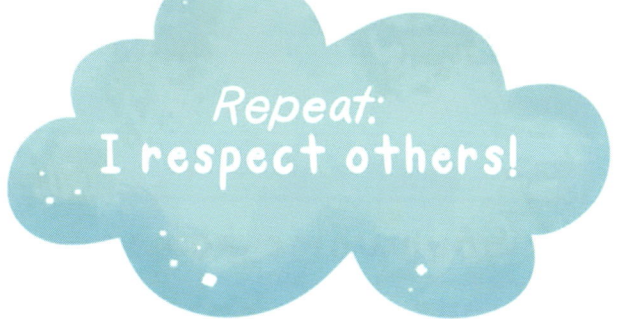

Know your boundaries!
Talk about your boundaries!
Listen to others!

We all have a voice! Our voice belongs to us!

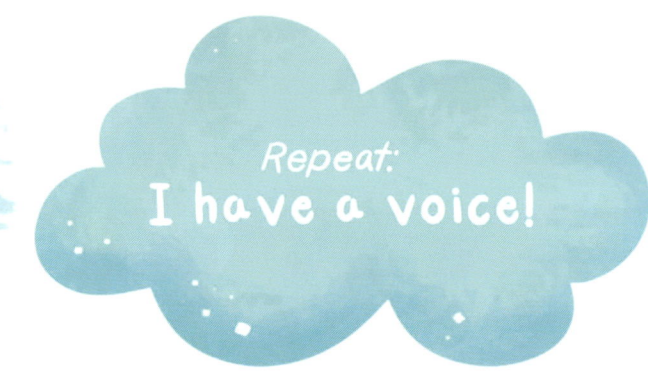

Repeat:
I have a voice!

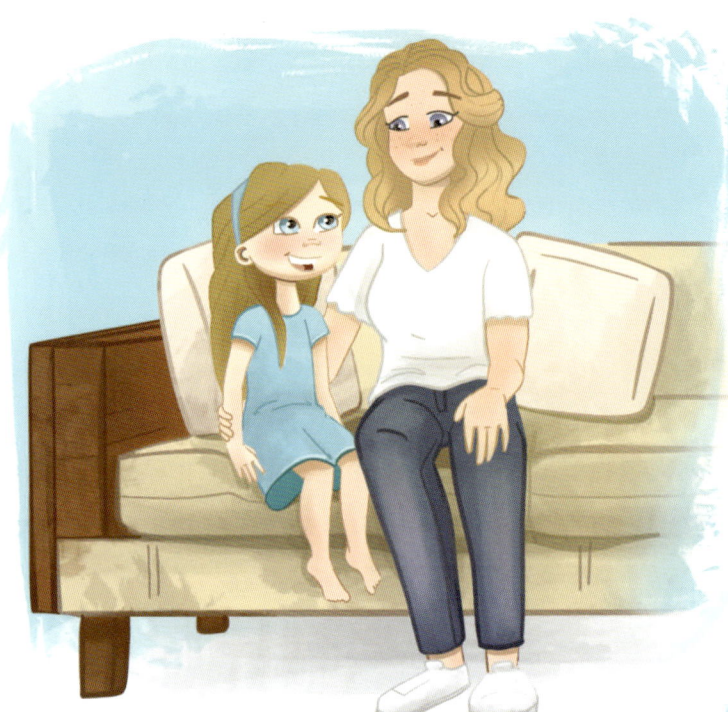

Use your voice to express your thoughts, concerns, and emotions.

Use your voice to ask questions. This book is a great reference that you can use any time!

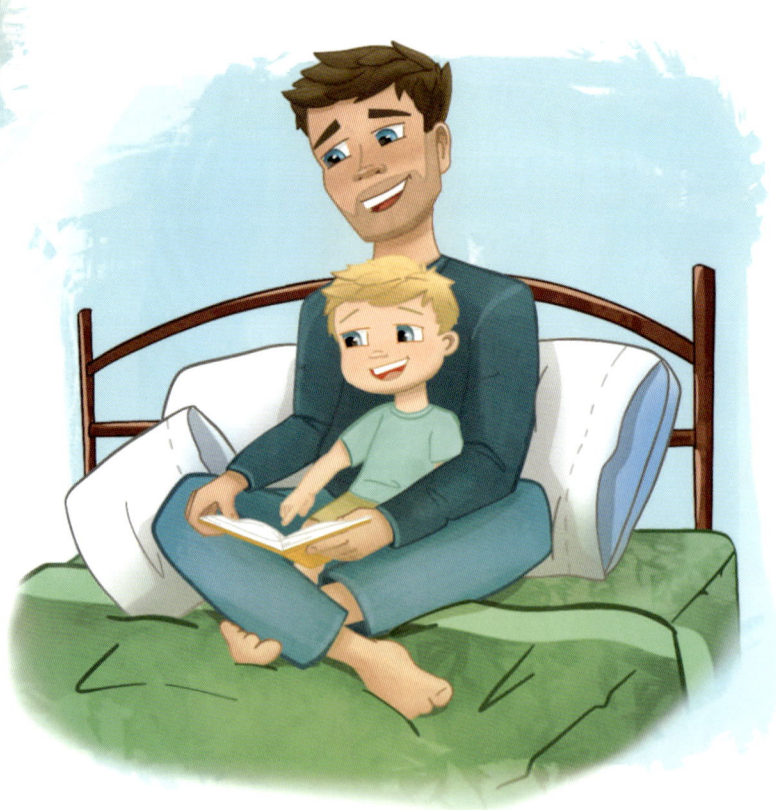

When you are in situations that feel uncomfortable, unsure, or unsafe, use your voice! Stand up for yourself! Say no! Walk or run away! Yell! Find and tell a trusted adult!

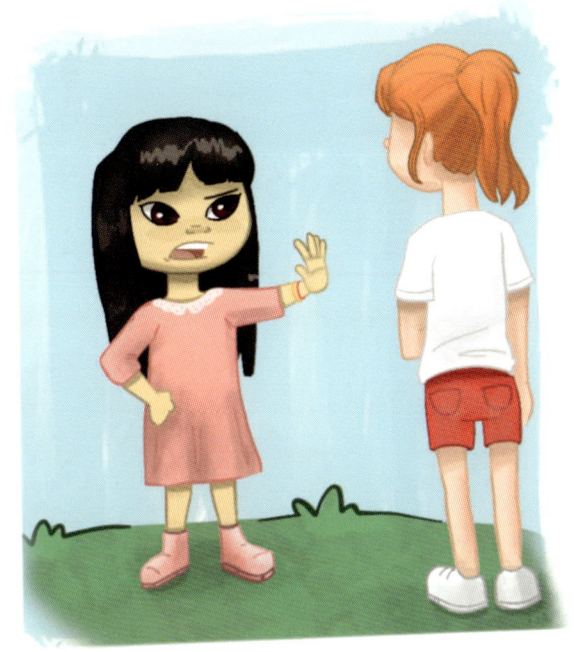

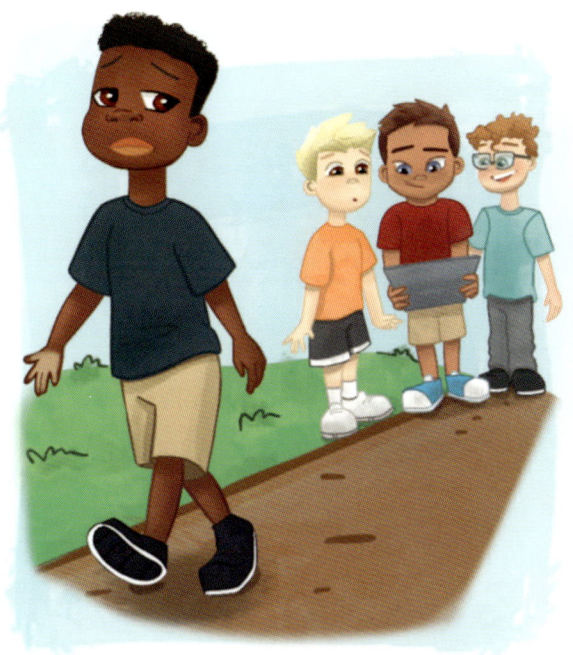

Even if you can't say no at the time, always tell a trusted adult. Keep telling until someone believes you!

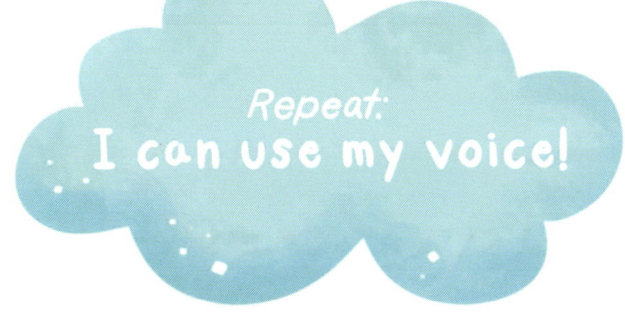

Repeat:
I can use my voice!

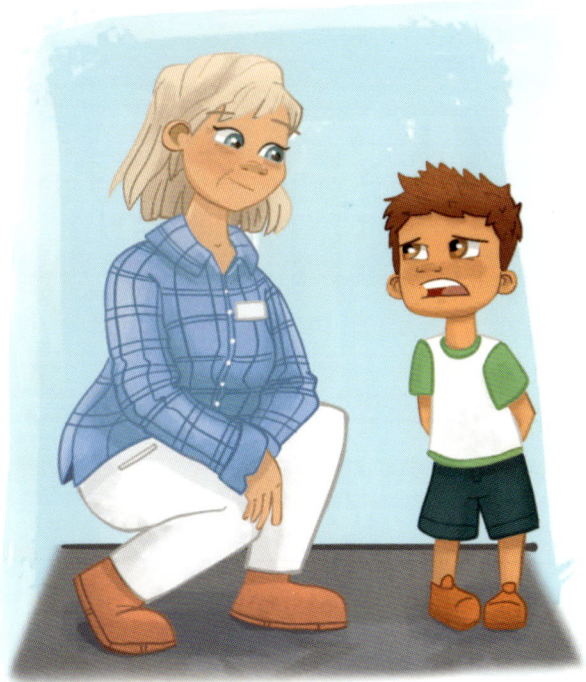

We don't keep secrets. If someone tells you to keep a secret, tell a trusted adult.

THIRD...

It is important to know how to love and take care of ourselves!

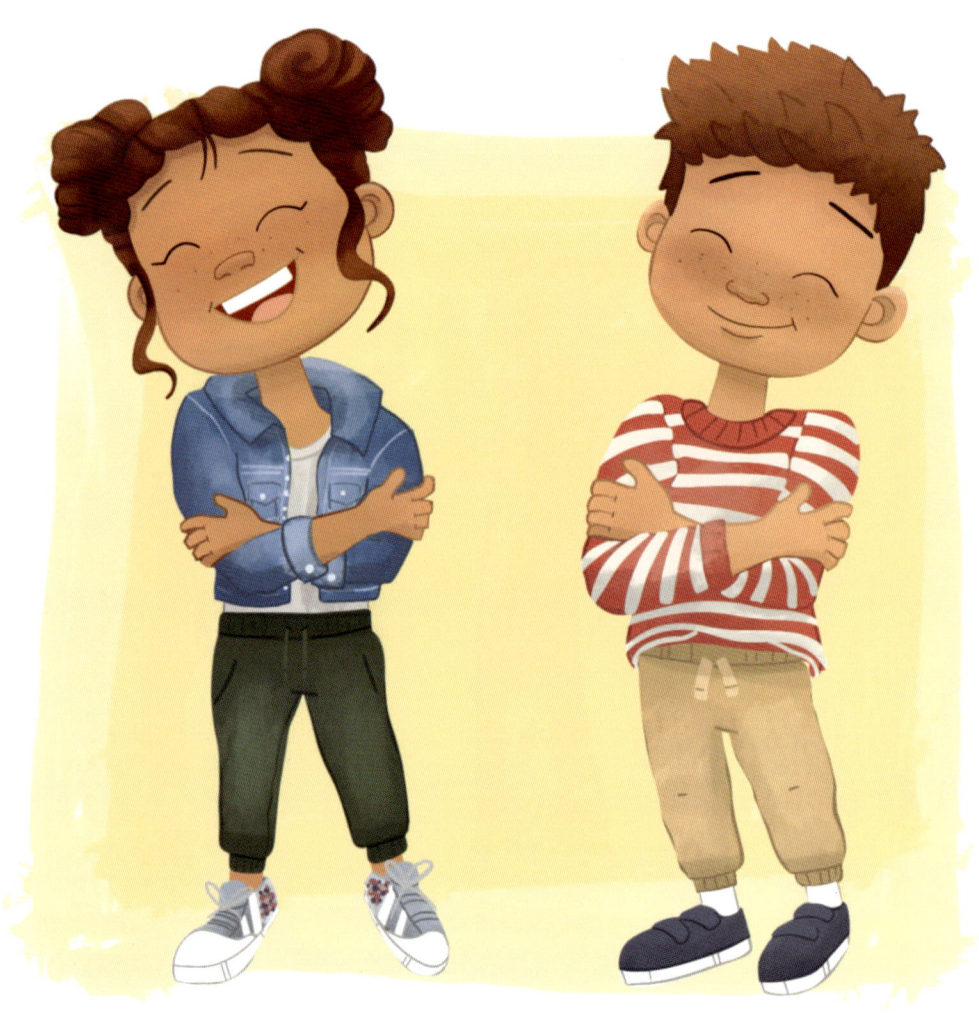

The next pages show ways to practice self-care.

We can practice self-care by expressing gratitude! Write, draw, or say three new things that you are grateful for every day.

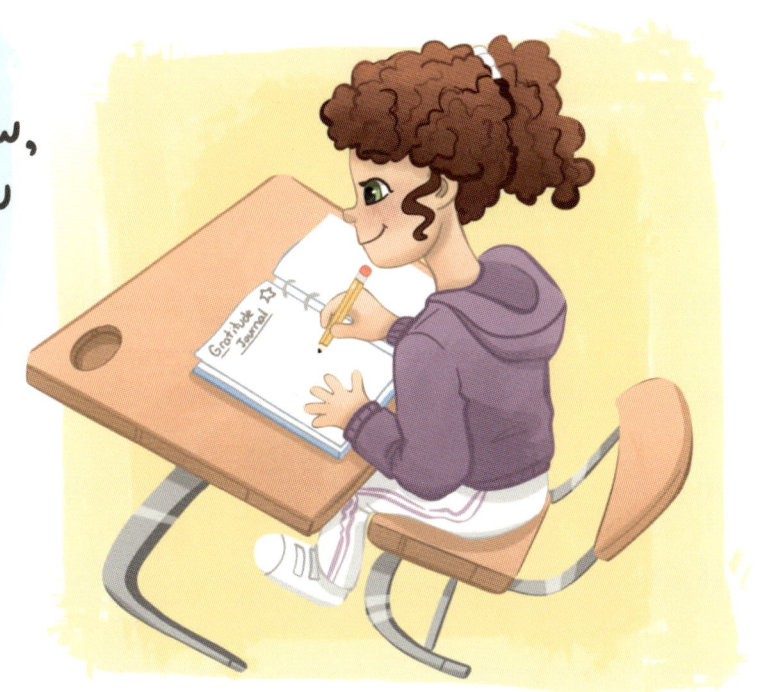

Repeat:
I am grateful!
I can practice gratitude every day!

What are you grateful for?

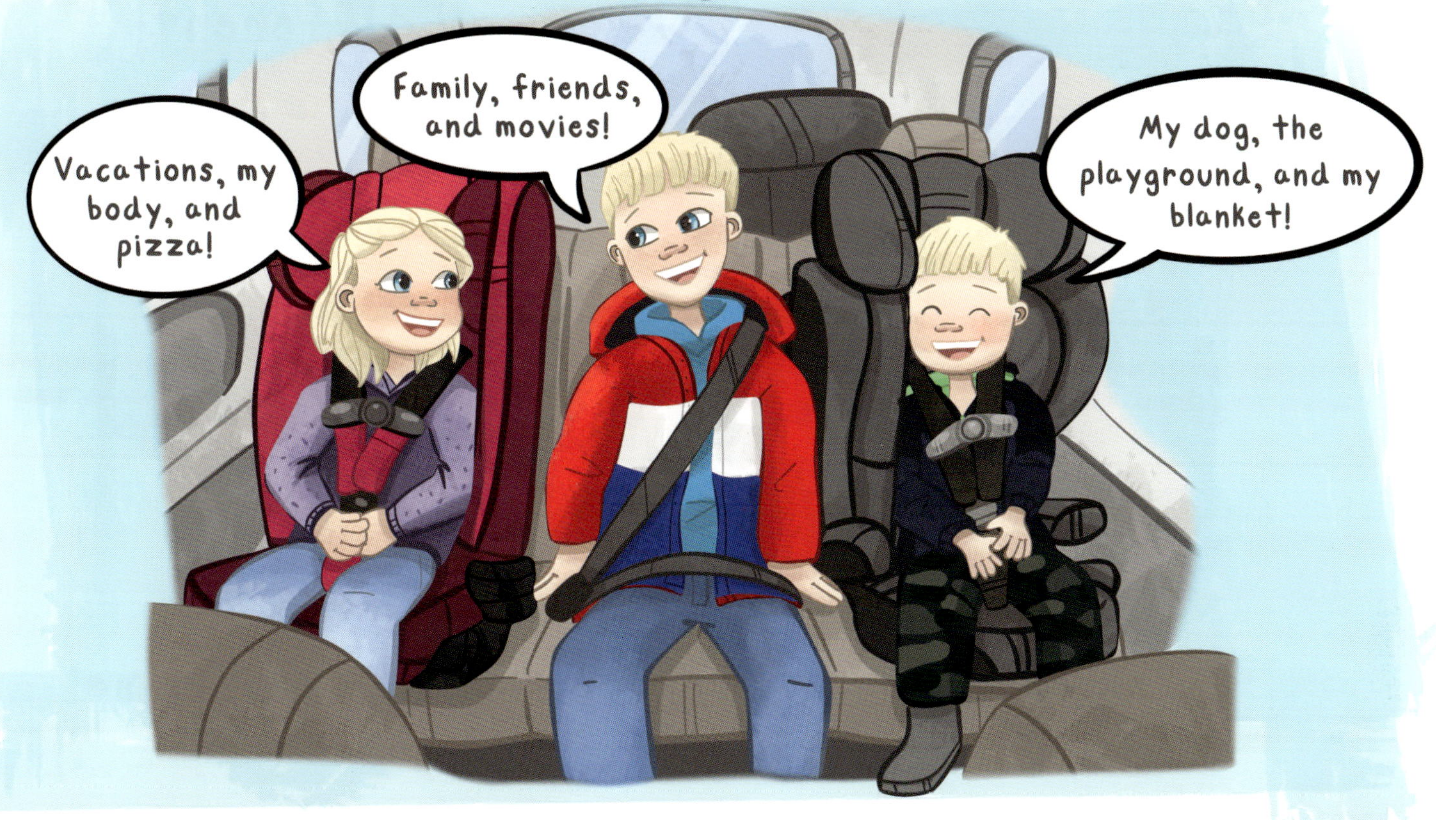

Vacations, my body, and pizza!

Family, friends, and movies!

My dog, the playground, and my blanket!

We can practice self-care by being confident! We can be confident by thinking good things about ourselves!

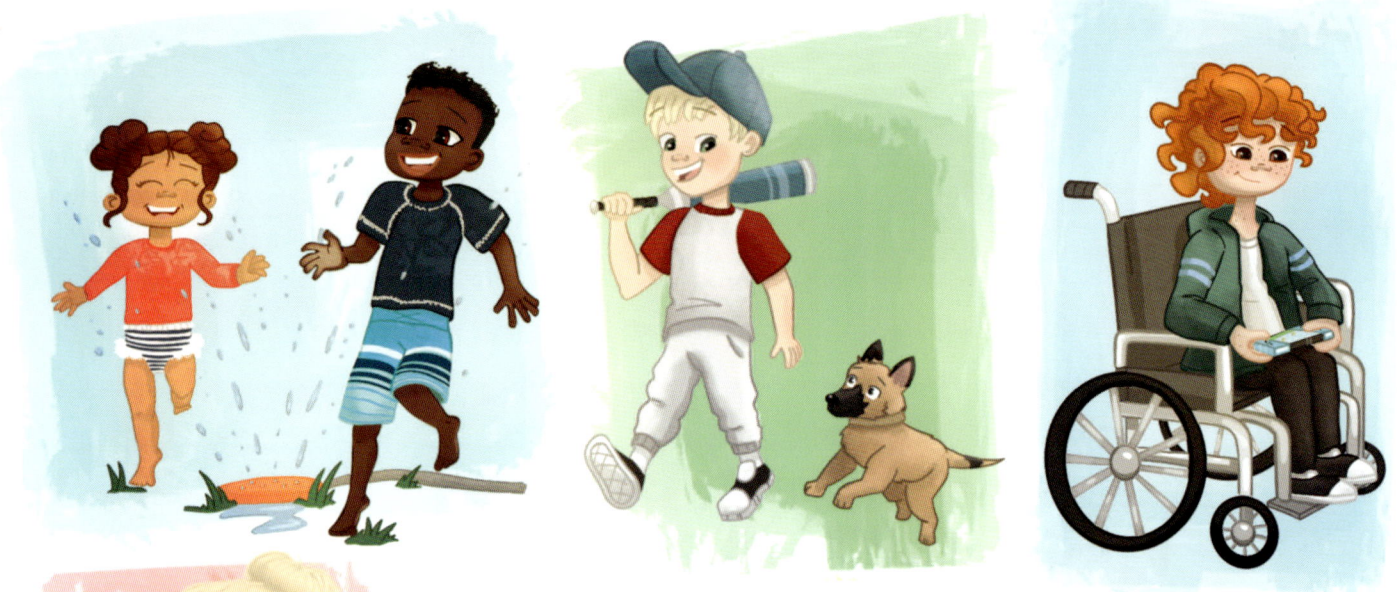

We are all different!

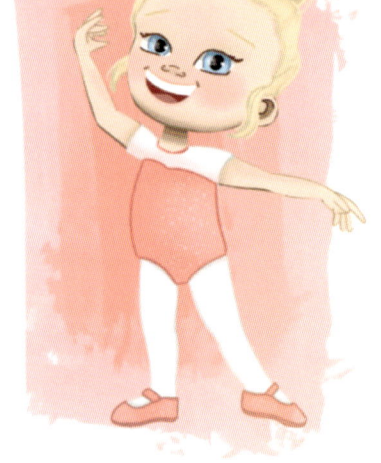

Repeat:
I am confident!

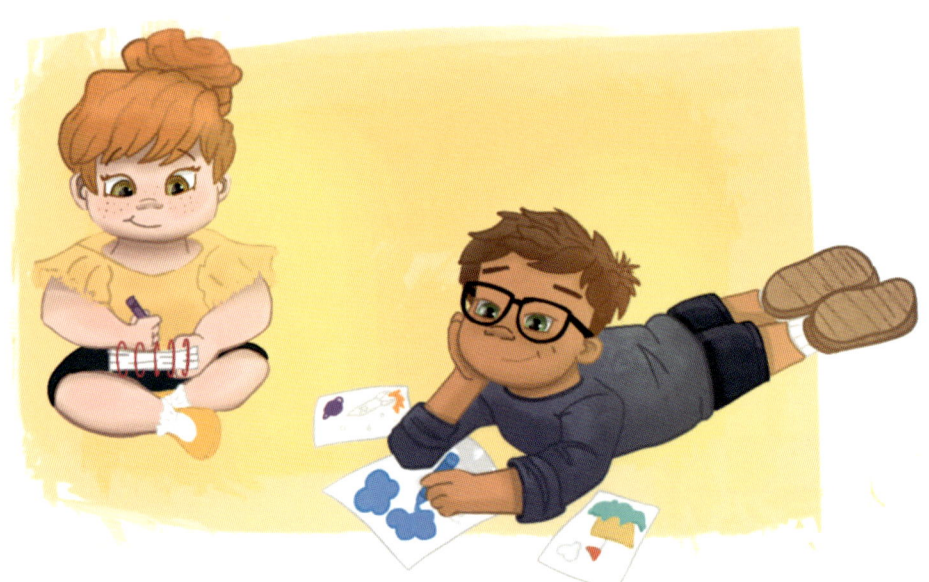

Differences are awesome!

We look different!

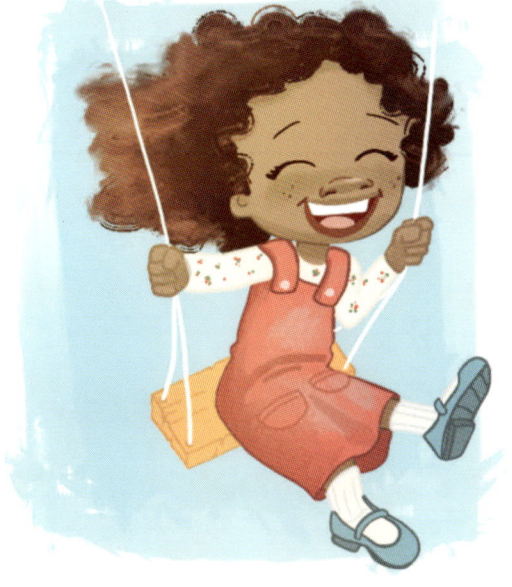

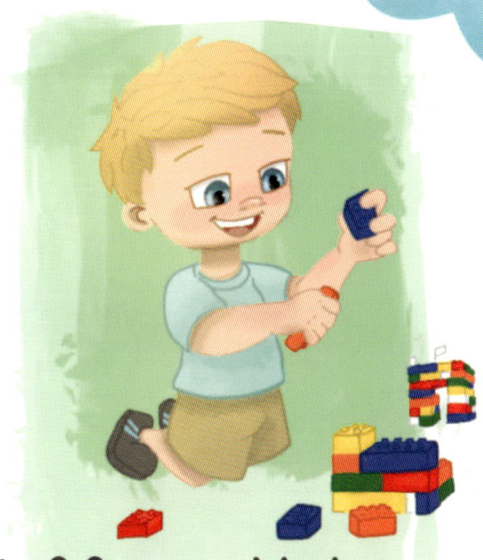

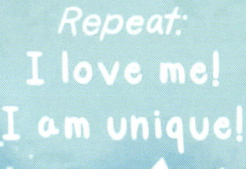
Repeat:
I love me!
I am unique!

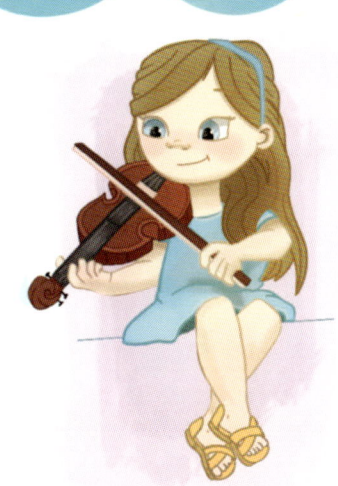

We think differently!

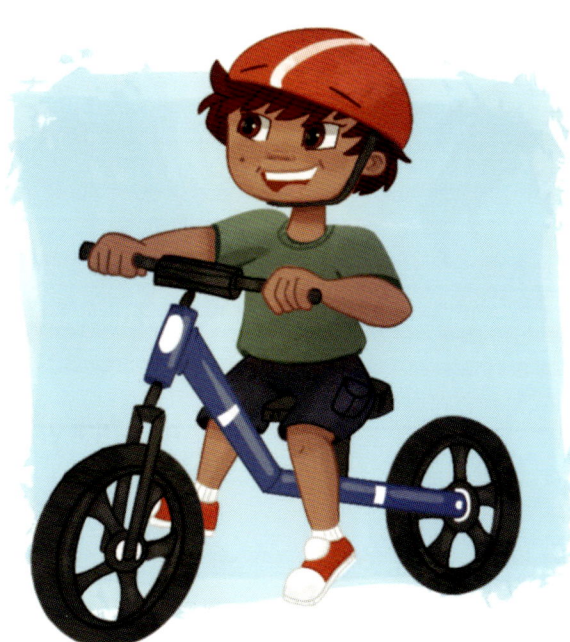

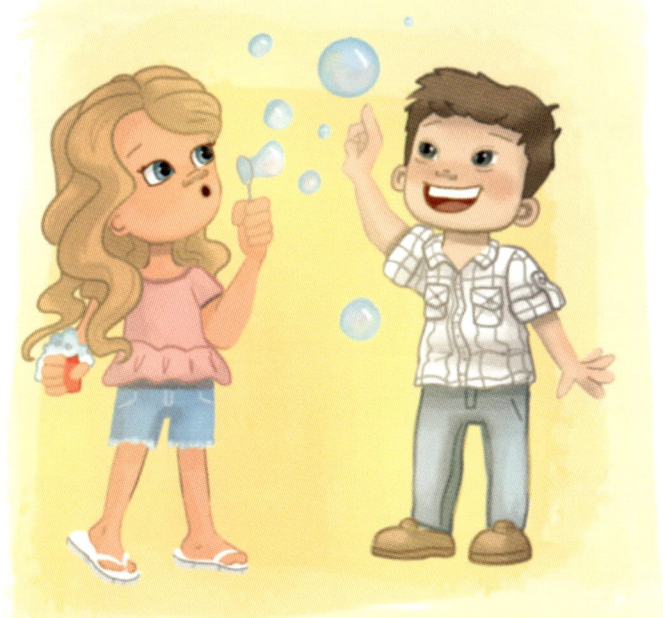

We like different things!

We can do things every day to help keep our bodies healthy, clean, and strong!

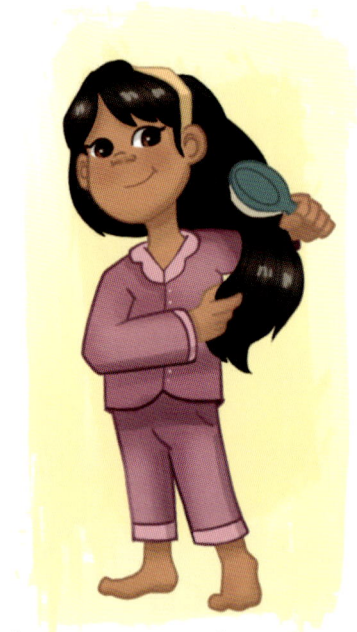

Repeat:
My body is important!

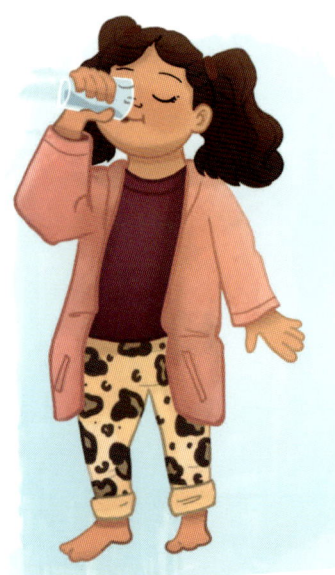

Drinking water!

Brushing or combing your hair!

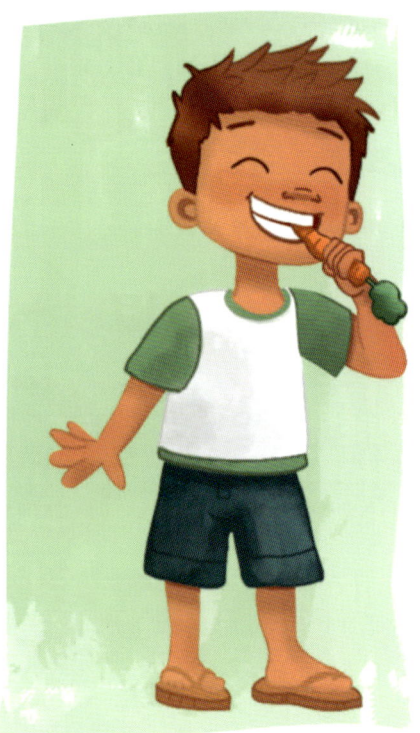

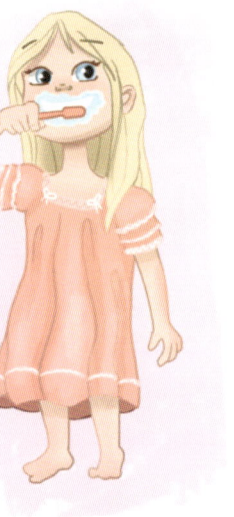

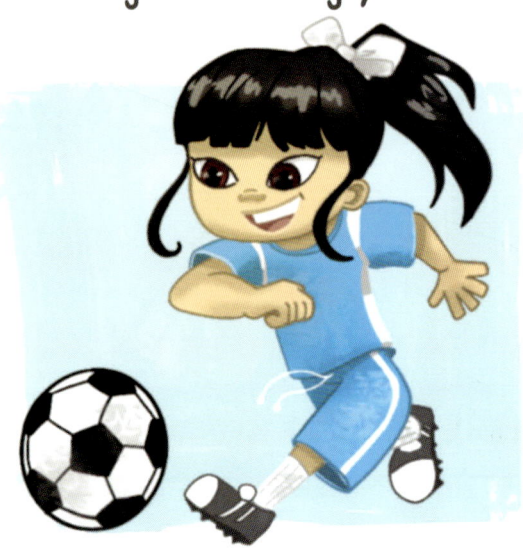

Brushing your teeth!

Moving your body!

Eating healthy foods!

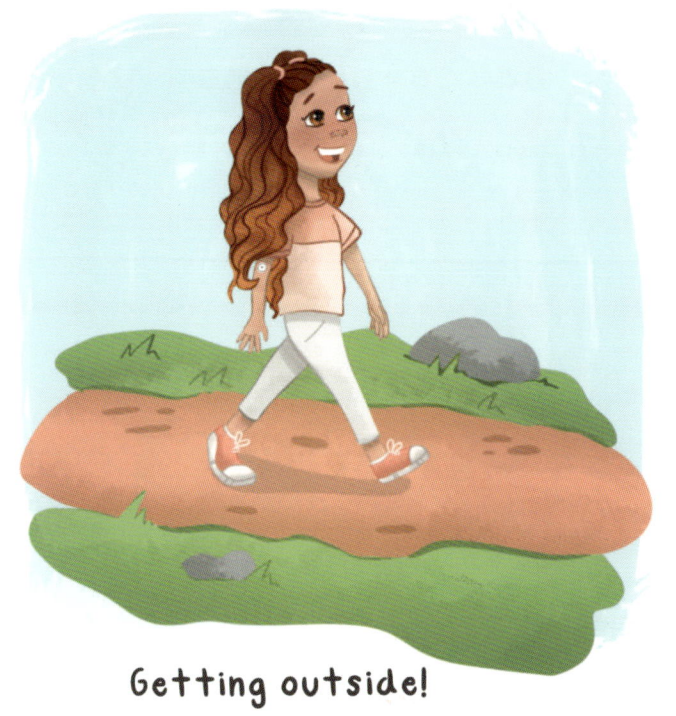

Getting outside!

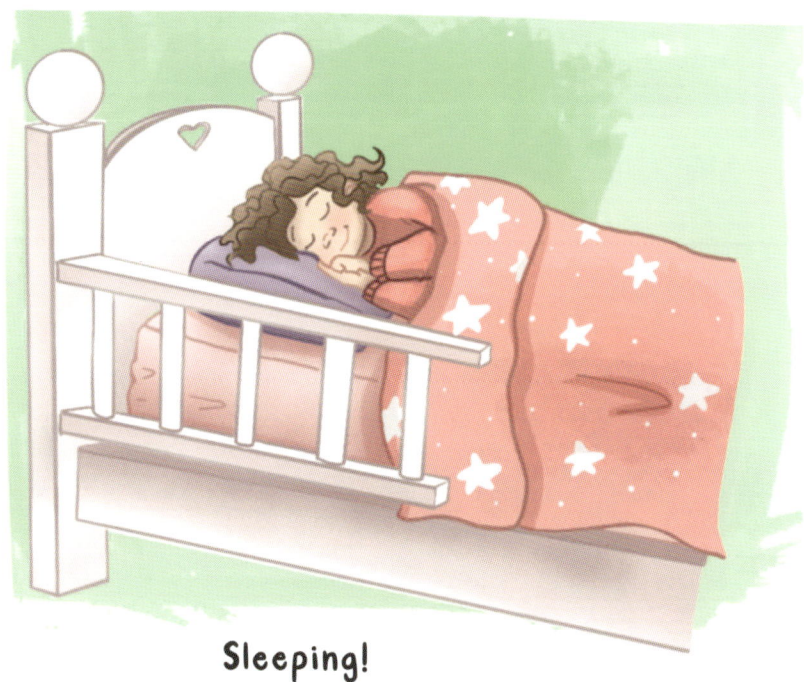

Sleeping!

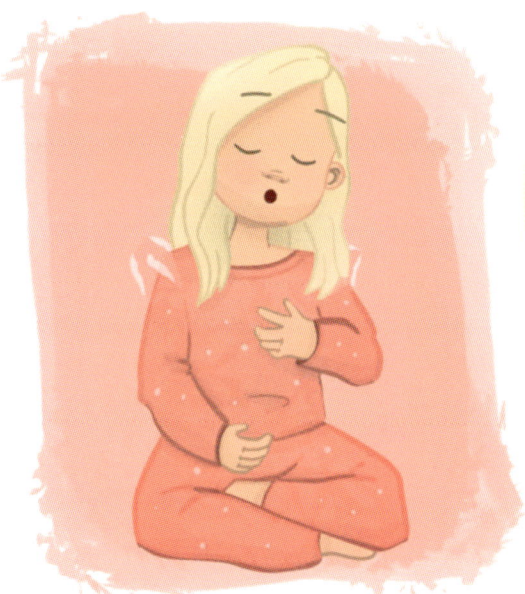

Taking deep breaths!

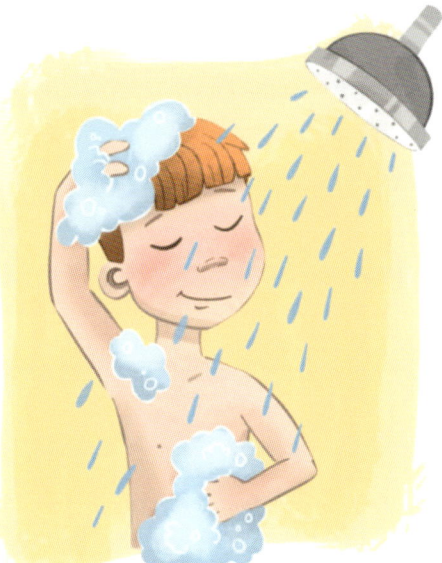

Washing your body!

Repeat:
I love my body!
I can take care of my body
every day!

We can do things every day to help us feel happy, peaceful, creative, and connected with others!

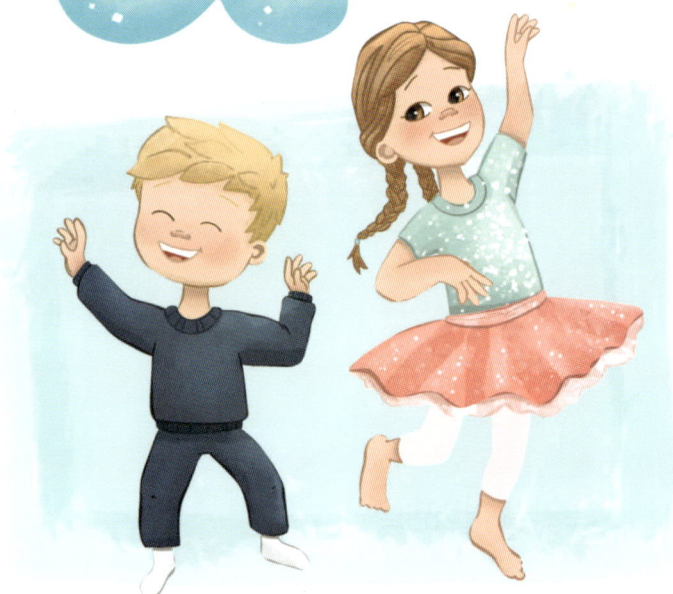

Joyful movement!

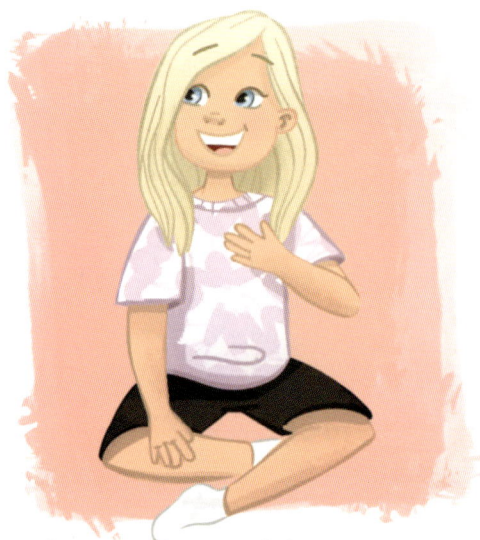

Repeating affirmations!

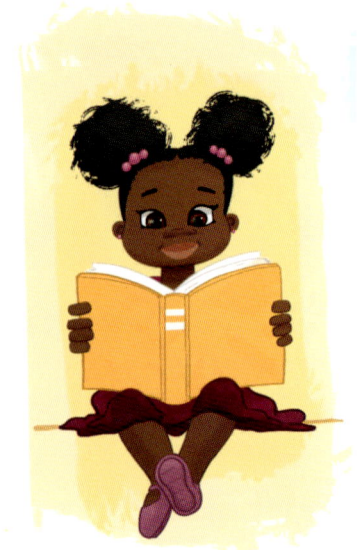

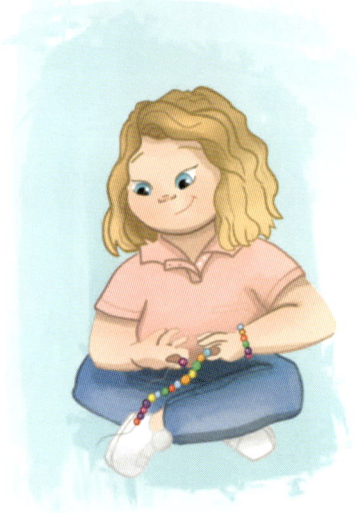

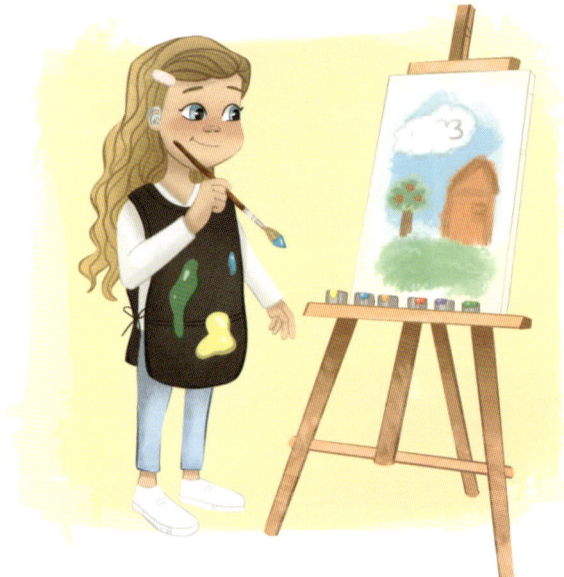

Reading, art, hobbies, and crafts!

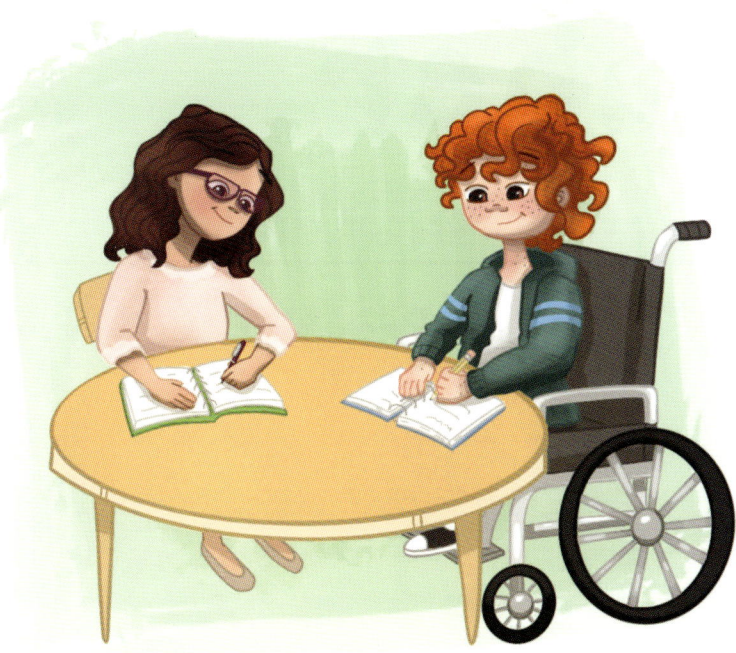

Writing or drawing your thoughts and feelings!

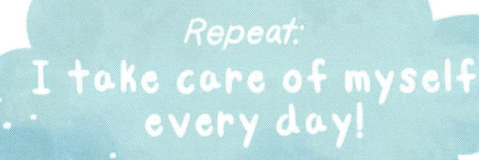

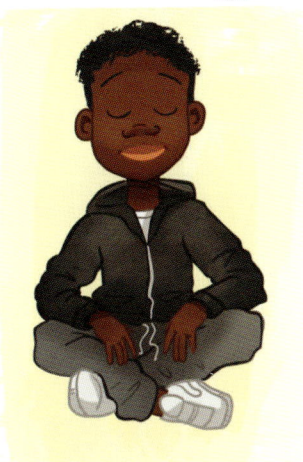

Meditating!

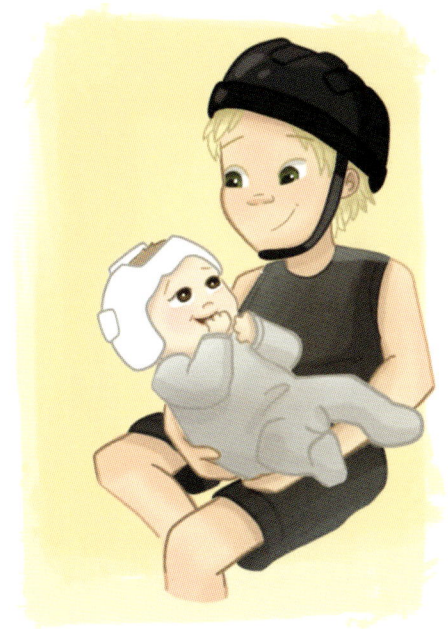

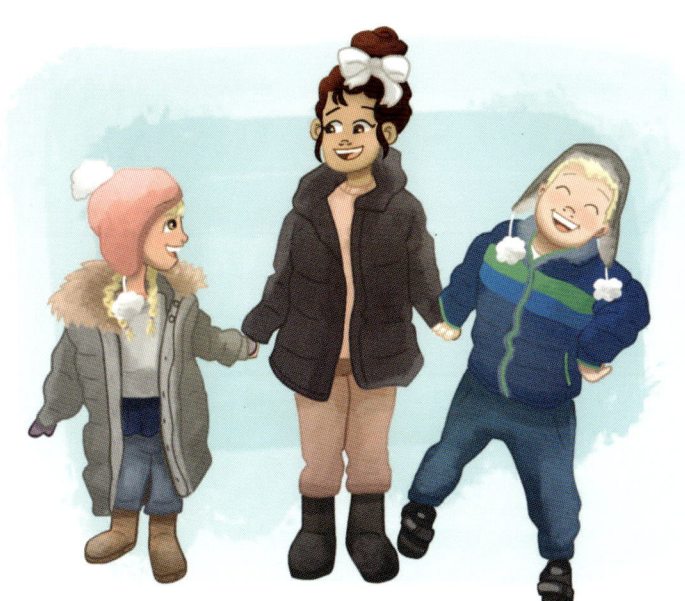

Connecting with others!

Remember...

Repeat affirmations!

Practice confidence!

Use proper names for your body parts!

Practice self-care!

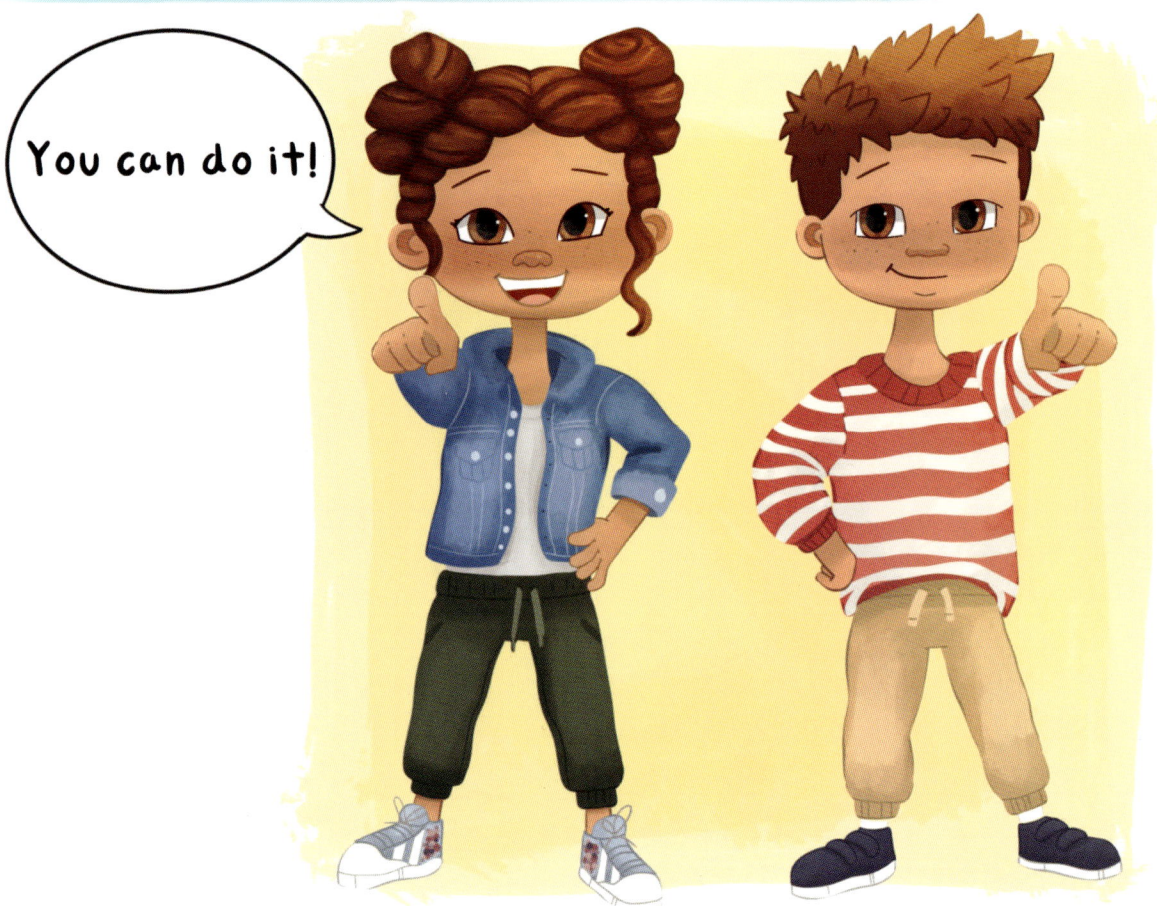

Let a safe adult help!

Take care of your body!

Practice gratitude everyday!

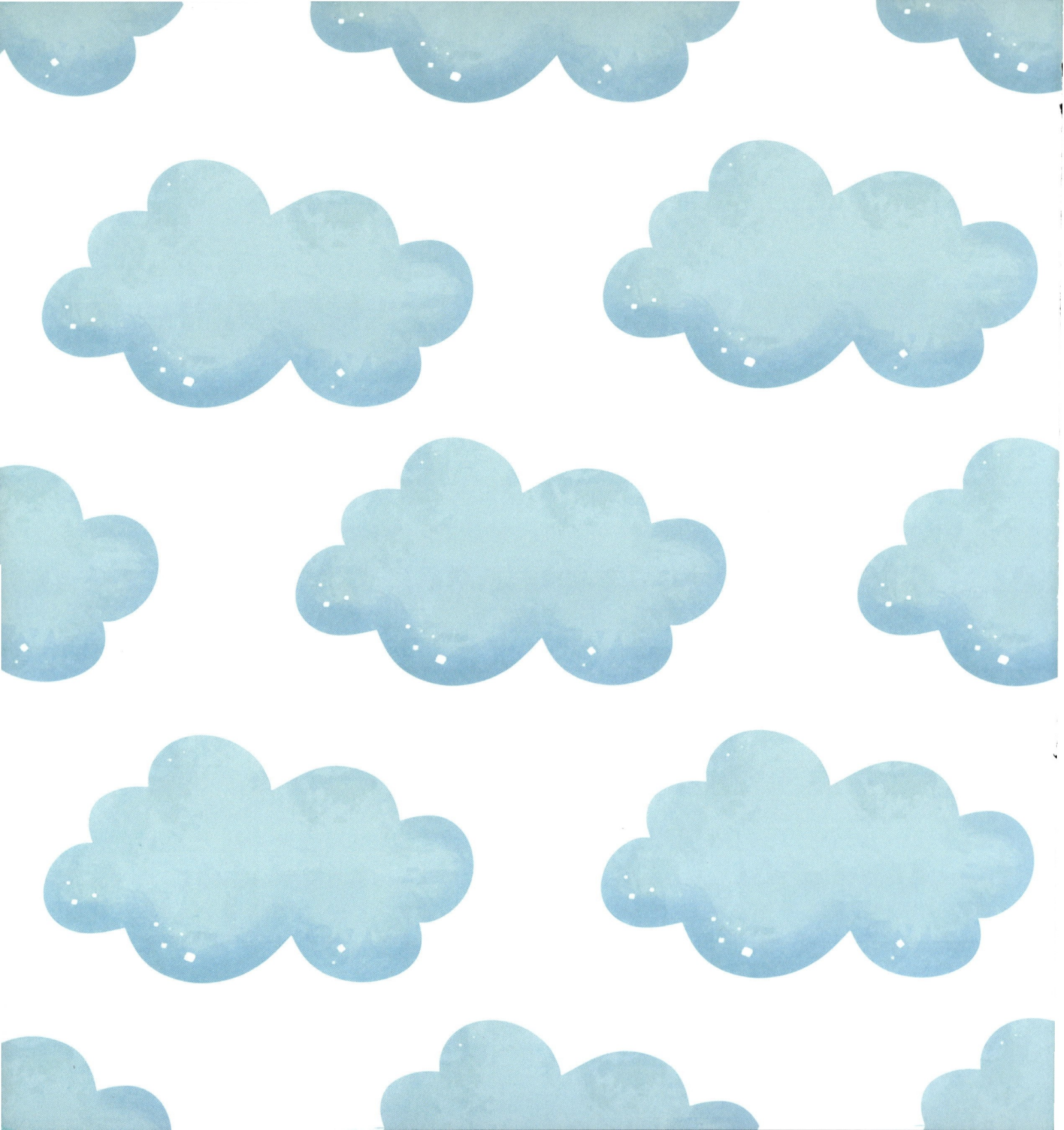